ICD-10-CM

Coding Excellence Workbook

Guidelines, Video Course & Medical Case Studies for Coding Success

Rory George

EXCLUSIVE LEARNING EXTRAS FOR YOU!

(See the last chapter)

DIGITAL COPY OF THIS BOOK to have with you at all times for revision whenever and wherever you want.

DIRECT CONTACT for assistance or clarifications, ensuring continuous support in your preparation.

COMPLETE VIDEO COURSE: Dive deeper into essential topics like ICD-10-CM coding, medical billing errors, and revenue cycle processes through a professionally designed video course tailored for medical coding professionals specializing in diagnosis coding.

3000 MEDICAL TERMS FLASHCARDS:

- **2500 Medical Terms** covering Surgery, Emergency Medicine, and Anesthesiology.
- **50 Flashcards featuring Real-World Case Studies** illustrating medical conditions and treatments for practical application in billing and coding.
- **600 Medical Terms** *with pictures*

Both are available in **PDF format** (ready to print) and **.APKG format** for the **Anki app**, allowing for a dynamic and interactive study experience.

💡 **Compatible with:**
✓ Anki App (iOS)
✓ AnkiDroid (Android)
✓ AnkiWeb (browser-based for desktop & mobile)
✓ Anki (PC & Mac)

⬇ **Instant Download:** Access the flashcards directly from our website—no registration or payment required. Simply import them into your preferred app and start studying at your own pace while tracking your progress.

EXTRA RESOURCE OF YOUR CHOICE: Select one additional resource to enhance your learning journey:

- *Medical Billing and Coding Study Guide*
- *CPC Study Guide*
- *CPT Professional Mastery Workbook*
- *HCPCS Level II Coding Workbook*

more details in the last chapter!

TABLE OF CONTENTS

WELCOME TO MEDICAL CODING MASTERY

This workbook is designed to help students to develop a solid understanding of ICD-10-CM coding. It provides structured exercises, real-world scenarios, and clear explanations to reinforce key coding principles.

Medical coding requires accuracy, attention to detail, and a strong grasp of coding guidelines. This workbook serves as a practical resource for mastering the ICD-10-CM classification system, ensuring compliance with official standards.

By working through this book, students will:

- Gain hands-on experience with ICD-10-CM coding conventions and guidelines.
- Improve accuracy in assigning diagnosis codes.
- Learn best practices to avoid common coding errors.
- Prepare effectively for the medical coding certification exams (such as CPC, CCS) through targeted exercises.

Each section builds progressively, offering a step-by-step approach to mastering medical coding. Whether you're new to coding or refining your skills, this workbook provides the structured learning needed for exam success and real-world application.

'Overview of ICD-10-CM Coding'

ICD-10-CM is the standardized system used in the United States for coding medical diagnoses. It is maintained by the National Center for Health Statistics (NCHS) and follows the guidelines set by the World Health Organization (WHO). This system ensures uniform documentation of diseases, conditions, and health-related issues across healthcare settings.

ICD-10-CM codes are alphanumeric and organized into chapters based on different body systems and conditions. Each code provides detailed information about a patient's diagnosis, supporting accurate medical records, billing, and statistical analysis.

Understanding how to use ICD-10-CM correctly is essential for medical coders, as it impacts reimbursement, compliance, and overall healthcare data quality. This workbook introduces the foundational concepts needed to apply ICD-10-CM coding effectively.

'Introduction to the Basic Principles and Coding System'

'Structure of ICD-10-CM'

The International Classification of Diseases, 10th Revision, Clinical Modification (ICD-10-CM) is a comprehensive system used in the United States for coding various medical diagnoses. It consists of alphanumeric codes, each starting with a letter followed by up to six digits, allowing for detailed classification of diseases and health conditions. The system is organized into 21 chapters, each focusing on a specific body system or medical condition, facilitating precise documentation and analysis.

'Code Composition'

Each ICD-10-CM code provides specific information about a diagnosis:

- **First Character**: Denotes the chapter or body system (e.g., 'A' for infectious diseases).
- **Second and Third Characters**: Represent the category of the disease.
- **Fourth to Sixth Characters**: Offer additional details such as etiology, anatomical site, and severity.
- **Seventh Character**: Used in certain chapters to indicate encounter type or disease sequelae.

This structured format ensures that each code conveys comprehensive information about the patient's condition.

'Recent Updates and Revisions'

As of October 1, 2024, the ICD-10-CM system has undergone significant updates to enhance specificity and accuracy in medical coding. These changes include the addition of 252 new codes, the deletion of 36 obsolete codes, and the revision of 13 existing ones. Notable updates encompass expanded codes for lymphoma classifications, refined definitions for eating disorders, and new codes addressing social determinants of health, such as insufficient insurance coverage. These modifications aim to improve the precision of medical documentation and ensure alignment with current clinical practices.

'Importance of Accurate Coding'

Proficient use of the ICD-10-CM coding system is essential for several reasons:

- **'Reimbursement'**: Ensures healthcare providers receive appropriate payment for services rendered.
- **'Compliance'**: Meets legal and regulatory requirements, reducing the risk of audits and penalties.
- **'Data Quality'**: Contributes to reliable health statistics and research.
- **'Patient Care'**: Facilitates effective communication among healthcare providers, leading to improved patient outcomes.

Understanding and applying the basic principles of the ICD-10-CM coding system is crucial for accurate medical documentation, efficient billing processes, and high-quality patient care.

Coding Terms and Definitions

Coding Term	Definition
Alphabetic Index	A list of diseases, conditions, and external causes arranged alphabetically with corresponding ICD-10-CM codes.
Tabular List	A structured list of ICD-10-CM codes organized by chapter and category based on body systems and conditions.
Placeholder Character (X)	A character used within some ICD-10-CM codes to maintain the correct code structure when additional characters are required.
Laterality	Specifies the affected side of the body (e.g., right, left, bilateral).
Combination Code	A single code that represents two or more conditions or a condition with an associated complication.
Sequela	A condition that results from a previous disease or injury, requiring a special code to indicate its relationship.
Excludes1 Note	A guideline indicating that two conditions cannot be coded together because they describe different conditions.
Excludes2 Note	A guideline that means the condition listed is not part of the main diagnosis but could be reported separately if applicable.
Primary Diagnosis	The main condition that is chiefly responsible for the patient's visit or treatment.
Secondary Diagnosis	Additional conditions that coexist or affect patient care but are not the primary reason for the visit.

FOUNDATIONS OF ICD-10-CM

The International Classification of Diseases, 10th Revision, Clinical Modification (ICD-10-CM) is a comprehensive coding system used in the United States to classify and code all diagnoses, symptoms, and procedures recorded in conjunction with hospital care. Developed by the Centers for Disease Control and Prevention's National Center for Health Statistics (NCHS), ICD-10-CM enhances the specificity and detail of health-related data, facilitating improved patient care and streamlined healthcare administration.

ICD-10-CM is structured to provide detailed information about a patient's condition, supporting accurate documentation and efficient healthcare delivery. The system is regularly updated to reflect advancements in medical knowledge and technology. For instance, the fiscal year 2025 update, effective from October 1, 2024, introduced 252 new codes, revised 36 existing ones, and deleted 13 obsolete codes. These updates ensure that the coding system remains current with evolving medical practices and emerging health concerns.

Understanding the foundational principles of ICD-10-CM is essential for healthcare professionals, particularly those preparing for the Certified Professional Coder (CPC) exam. Proficiency in this coding system ensures accurate reporting of patient diagnoses and procedures, which is critical for effective communication among healthcare providers, appropriate reimbursement, and the generation of reliable health statistics.

This chapter provides an overview of the basic structure and principles of ICD-10-CM, laying the groundwork for more advanced coding practices discussed in subsequent sections.

Structure and Format

The International Classification of Diseases, 10th Revision, Clinical Modification (ICD-10-CM) is a comprehensive coding system used in the United States to classify and code medical diagnoses. Its structure and format are designed to provide detailed and specific information about a patient's condition, facilitating accurate documentation and efficient healthcare delivery.

'Code Composition'

ICD-10-CM codes are alphanumeric and can range from three to seven characters in length. The first character is always a letter, which indicates the chapter or body system. The second and third characters are numbers that define the category of the diagnosis. Characters four through six, which can be either letters or numbers, provide additional details such as etiology, anatomic site, and severity. A seventh character, when applicable, serves as an extension to convey information about the encounter type or sequelae. For example, in injury codes, the seventh character distinguishes between initial encounters, subsequent encounters, or sequelae.

'Placeholder Character'

To accommodate future code expansion and ensure code validity, ICD-10-CM utilizes a placeholder character 'X'. This character is used in certain codes to fill empty positions when a code requires a seventh character but does not have enough characters to reach that length. For instance, if a code has only four characters and requires a seventh character, 'X' is used to fill the fifth and sixth positions.

'Laterality'

One of the enhancements in ICD-10-CM over its predecessors is the inclusion of laterality. Many codes specify whether the condition occurs on the left side, right side, or is bilateral. This specificity improves the accuracy of clinical data and ensures precise communication among healthcare providers.

'Updates and Revisions'

ICD-10-CM is regularly updated to reflect advancements in medical knowledge and practice. The National Center for Health Statistics (NCHS) releases annual updates to the coding guidelines and code sets. These updates may include the addition of new codes, revisions to existing codes, and deletions of obsolete codes. Staying informed about these changes is essential for accurate coding and compliance.

Understanding the structure and format of ICD-10-CM is fundamental for medical coders, healthcare providers, and students preparing for certification exams. Proficiency in navigating and applying this coding system ensures precise documentation, effective communication, and optimal patient care.

Anatomy of the ICD-10-CM Code

The International Classification of Diseases, 10th Revision, Clinical Modification (ICD-10-CM) is a comprehensive coding system used in the United States to classify and code medical diagnoses. Each ICD-10-CM code provides detailed information about a patient's condition, facilitating accurate documentation and efficient healthcare delivery.

'Structure of ICD-10-CM Codes'

ICD-10-CM codes are alphanumeric and can range from three to seven characters in length. The structure of these codes is designed to convey specific information about the diagnosis:

- **'First Character'**: Always a letter, indicating the chapter or body system.
- **'Second and Third Characters'**: Numbers that define the category of the diagnosis.
- **'Fourth to Sixth Characters'**: Alphanumeric characters providing additional details such as etiology, anatomic site, and severity.
- **'Seventh Character'**: When applicable, this character serves as an extension to convey information about the encounter type or sequel.

For example, the code **S52.521A** represents a torus fracture of the lower end of the right radius, initial encounter. Here, 'S' denotes an injury, '52' specifies the forearm, '5' indicates a fracture of the lower end of the radius, '2' specifies a torus fracture, '1' denotes the right side, and 'A' signifies an initial encounter.

Placeholder Character 'X'

To ensure the code maintains the correct length and structure, ICD-10-CM utilizes a placeholder character 'X'. This character is used in certain codes to fill empty positions when a code requires a seventh character but does not have enough characters to reach that length. For instance, in the code **W04.XXXA** (fall while being carried or supported by other persons, initial encounter), 'XXX' serves as placeholders to allow for the seventh character 'A'.

'Laterality'

ICD-10-CM includes the concept of laterality, allowing coders to specify whether a condition affects the left side, right side, or is bilateral. This specificity enhances the accuracy of clinical data and ensures precise communication among healthcare providers. For example, the codes **H16.011** and **H16.012** denote central corneal ulcer of the right eye and left eye, respectively.

Importance of Detailed Coding

Accurate and detailed ICD-10-CM coding is essential for several reasons:

- **Reimbursement**: Ensures healthcare providers receive appropriate payment for services rendered.
- **Compliance**: Meets legal and regulatory requirements, reducing the risk of audits and penalties.
- **Data Quality**: Contributes to reliable health statistics and research.
- **Patient Care**: Facilitates effective communication among healthcare providers, leading to improved patient outcomes.

Understanding the anatomy of ICD-10-CM codes enables medical coders and healthcare professionals to accurately capture patient diagnoses, supporting effective treatment plans and contributing to the overall efficiency of the healthcare system.

Fill-in-the-Blanks Activity: Identify Components of Sample ICD-10-CM Codes

Review the sample ICD-10-CM codes below and fill in the blanks to identify each component of the code. This activity reinforces an understanding of how ICD-10-CM codes are structured and applied.

1. **S72.001A** – _____ injury of _____, _____ encounter.
2. **I10** – Essential _____.
3. **E11.9** – Type _____ diabetes mellitus without _____.
4. **J18.9** – _____, unspecified.
5. **M54.5** – _____ pain.
6. **H25.11** – _____ cataract, _____ eye.
7. **W19.XXXA** – Unspecified _____, _____ encounter.
8. **G40.909** – Epilepsy, _____ type, _____ side.
9. **L89.312** – Pressure ulcer of _____, stage _____.
10. **T14.90XA** – _____ injury, unspecified, _____ encounter.

Answer Key for Structure and Format

1. S72.001A – Fracture injury of right femur, initial encounter.
2. I10 – Essential hypertension.
3. E11.9 – Type 2 diabetes mellitus without complications.
4. J18.9 – Pneumonia, unspecified.
5. M54.5 – Low back pain.
6. H25.11 – Age-related cataract, right eye.
7. W19.XXXA – Unspecified fall, initial encounter.
8. G40.909 – Epilepsy, unspecified type, unspecified side.
9. L89.312 – Pressure ulcer of right buttock, stage 2.
10. T14.90XA – Unspecified injury, unspecified, initial encounter.

Coding Guidelines

The ICD-10-CM **Official Guidelines for Coding and Reporting** are essential instructions developed by the Centers for Medicare & Medicaid Services (CMS) and the National Center for Health Statistics (NCHS). These guidelines, updated annually, provide standardized directions for coding and reporting diagnoses across all healthcare settings in the United States. Adherence to these guidelines ensures consistency, accuracy, and compliance in medical documentation and billing. The latest version, effective from October 1, 2024, reflects the most recent updates and revisions in medical coding practices.

The guidelines are organized into several sections:

- **'Section I'**: Conventions, general coding guidelines, and chapter-specific guidelines.
- **'Section II'**: Selection of principal diagnosis.
- **'Section III'**: Reporting additional diagnoses.
- **'Section IV'**: Diagnostic coding and reporting guidelines for outpatient services.

Each section addresses specific aspects of coding, providing detailed instructions to ensure accurate code assignment. For instance, Section I covers the structure and conventions of the classification system, while Section II offers guidance on selecting the principal diagnosis in various healthcare settings. These guidelines are integral to achieving complete and precise documentation, which is crucial for patient care, statistical analysis, and reimbursement processes.

Staying current with these guidelines is vital for healthcare professionals, as they reflect the latest medical knowledge and coding standards. Regular review and application of the most recent guidelines ensure that coding practices align with contemporary clinical practices and regulatory requirements. The FY 2025 updates, effective from October 1, 2024, include significant changes such as the introduction of new codes and revisions to existing ones, underscoring the dynamic nature of medical coding.

In summary, the ICD-10-CM Official Guidelines serve as a foundational resource for medical coders, healthcare providers, and compliance officers, guiding the accurate and consistent reporting of diagnoses across the healthcare continuum.

Essential Rules for Accurate Coding

Accurate medical coding is vital for effective healthcare management, impacting patient care, reimbursement, and compliance. The ICD-10-CM **Official Guidelines for Coding and Reporting** provide a framework to ensure consistency and precision in coding practices. Adhering to these guidelines is essential for all healthcare professionals involved in the coding process.

'Key Principles for Accurate Coding'

1. **'Use Current Codes and Guidelines'**
   - **'Annual Updates'**: The ICD-10-CM codes and guidelines are updated annually. For instance, the fiscal year 2025 updates, effective from October 1, 2024, introduced 252 new codes, revised 36 existing ones, and deleted 13 obsolete codes. Staying informed about these changes is crucial for maintaining coding accuracy.

2. **'Thorough Review of Medical Documentation'**
   - **'Comprehensive Analysis'**: Accurate coding begins with a detailed review of the patient's medical record, including history, examinations, test results, and provider notes. This ensures that all relevant diagnoses and procedures are captured.
   - **'Clarification When Needed'**: If documentation is unclear or incomplete, coders should seek clarification from the healthcare provider to ensure accurate code assignment.

3. **'Adherence to Coding Conventions and Instructions'**
   - **'Alphabetic Index and Tabular List'**: Utilize both the Alphabetic Index and the Tabular List when selecting codes. The Alphabetic Index assists in locating the appropriate code, which must then be verified in the Tabular List for accuracy.
   - **'Instructional Notes'**: Pay attention to notes such as "Includes," "Excludes1," "Excludes2," "Code first," and "Use additional code," as they provide critical guidance for correct coding.

4. **'Specificity and Detail in Coding'**
   - **'Highest Level of Specificity'**: Assign codes to the highest level of detail available, including laterality (right, left, bilateral) and specific anatomical locations. Codes with three characters are used only if no four-character codes exist for that condition.
   - **'Use of Placeholder 'X''**: In codes requiring a seventh character, but lacking six characters, the placeholder 'X' is used to fill the empty positions, ensuring the seventh character is in the correct position.

5. **'Sequencing of Codes'**
   - **'Principal Diagnosis'**: Identify and code the principal diagnosis first, which is the condition chiefly responsible for the patient's admission or encounter.
   - **'Secondary Diagnoses'**: List additional conditions that coexist or develop during the encounter and affect patient care or treatment.
   - **'Etiology and Manifestation'**: When coding conditions with an underlying cause and multiple manifestations, sequence the etiology (cause) code first, followed by the manifestation code. Instructional notes in the Tabular List provide guidance on proper sequencing.

6. **'Avoidance of Unspecified Codes'**
   - **'Detailed Documentation'**: Encourage providers to document with sufficient detail to allow for the most specific code assignment. While unspecified codes are available, their overuse can lead to issues with reimbursement and data quality.

7. **'Awareness of Excludes Notes'**
   - **'Excludes1 Note'**: Indicates that the excluded code should never be used at the same time as the code above the Excludes1 note, as the two conditions cannot occur together.
   - **'Excludes2 Note'**: Signifies that the excluded condition is not part of the condition represented by the code but may co-occur. It is acceptable to use both codes together if the patient has both conditions.

8. **'Application of Updated Coding Guidelines'**
   - **'Regular Review'**: Continuously review the latest ICD-10-CM guidelines to stay current with any changes or updates. The fiscal year 2025 guidelines, for example, include revisions to chapters on endocrine, nutritional, and metabolic diseases, among others.
   - **'Educational Resources'**: Utilize official resources, such as the Centers for Medicare & Medicaid Services (CMS) and the National Center for Health Statistics (NCHS), for authoritative information on coding practices.

Mastering the essential rules of accurate coding requires a commitment to ongoing education, meticulous attention to detail, and adherence to official guidelines. By implementing these principles, healthcare professionals can ensure precise documentation, optimal reimbursement, and high-quality patient care.

True/False Exercise: Test Your Understanding of the Coding Guidelines

'Instructions'

Read each statement carefully and determine whether it is **true** or **false** based on the latest ICD-10-CM coding guidelines.

'Statements'

1. The ICD-10-CM code set is updated every five years to reflect medical advancements.
2. Excludes1 notes mean that the listed conditions cannot be reported together under any circumstance.
3. A placeholder character "X" must be used when a code requires a seventh character but does not have enough characters.
4. The Alphabetic Index should always be used alone when assigning a code.
5. Laterality must be specified whenever applicable, indicating whether the condition affects the right, left, or both sides.
6. Principal diagnosis refers to the main condition that led to the patient's visit or admission.
7. Unspecified codes should always be used when a more specific code is available.
8. The seventh character in ICD-10-CM is only used for injury and poisoning codes.
9. Manifestation codes must always be sequenced before the underlying condition.
10. Coding guidelines are the same for inpatient and outpatient settings.

Exercise Challenge - Common Terminology

'Instructions'

Test your understanding of ICD-10-CM coding by completing the exercises below. Carefully analyze each scenario and select the most accurate code based on the given information.

'Part 1: Multiple-Choice Questions'

1. 'Which section of the ICD-10-CM guidelines provides instructions on selecting the principal diagnosis?'
   a) Section I
   b) Section II
   c) Section III
   d) Section IV
2. 'What does an Excludes1 note indicate?'
   a) The conditions can be coded together
   b) The conditions cannot be coded together under any circumstance
   c) The conditions are unrelated
   d) The condition is optional to report
3. 'What is the purpose of the placeholder character "X" in ICD-10-CM coding?'
   a) It is used as a wildcard to represent any number
   b) It is used in place of missing documentation
   c) It is used to fill empty positions when a seventh character is required
   d) It replaces unspecified codes

4. 'What does the seventh character in an injury code typically represent?'
   a) The severity of the injury
   b) Whether the injury is initial, subsequent, or a sequela
   c) The primary diagnosis
   d) The length of hospital stay
5. 'Laterality in ICD-10-CM refers to:'
   a) The type of condition being coded
   b) Whether the condition affects the right, left, or both sides of the body
   c) The anatomical location of the disease
   d) The coding sequence for injuries

'Part 2: Coding Scenarios'

Assign the correct ICD-10-CM code(s) for each of the following patient scenarios:

6. 'A 45-year-old male is diagnosed with type 2 diabetes mellitus without complications.
   ICD-10-CM **Code:** _____'
7. 'A patient is treated for a fracture of the right femur, initial encounter.
   ICD-10-CM **Code:** _____'
8. 'A 60-year-old woman presents with bilateral age-related cataracts.
   ICD-10-CM **Code:** _____'
9. 'A patient is seen for follow-up care for a healing pressure ulcer of the left heel, stage 3.
   ICD-10-CM **Code:** _____'
10. 'A child falls off playground equipment and suffers a concussion with loss of consciousness for less than 30 minutes. Initial encounter.
    ICD-10-CM **Code:** _____'

Answer Key for Coding Guidelines

1. **False** – The ICD-10-CM code set is updated annually, not every five years.
2. **True** – Excludes1 notes indicate that the two listed conditions cannot be coded together.
3. **True** – The placeholder "X" is used when a code requires a seventh character but lacks enough characters.
4. **False** – The Alphabetic Index should always be verified in the Tabular List before assigning a final code.
5. **True** – Laterality must be included when applicable, specifying right, left, or bilateral conditions.
6. **True** – The principal diagnosis is the main reason for the patient's visit or admission.
7. **False** – Unspecified codes should only be used when there is insufficient clinical documentation for a more specific code.
8. **False** – The seventh character is used in various code categories, including injuries, obstetric conditions, and musculoskeletal disorders.
9. **False** – Manifestation codes should be sequenced after the underlying condition, following coding guidelines.
10. **False** – Coding guidelines differ between inpatient and outpatient settings due to variations in reporting requirements.

Answer Key for Common Terminology

Part 1: Multiple-Choice Questions

1. **b) Section II** – This section provides instructions on selecting the principal diagnosis.
2. **b) The conditions cannot be coded together under any circumstance** – An Excludes1 note means two conditions should never be reported together.
3. **c) It is used to fill empty positions when a seventh character is required** – The placeholder "X" maintains the correct code structure.
4. **b) Whether the injury is initial, subsequent, or a sequela** – The seventh character in injury codes indicates encounter type.
5. **b) Whether the condition affects the right, left, or both sides of the body** – Laterality specifies which side of the body is affected.

Part 2: Coding Scenarios

6. **E11.9** – Type 2 diabetes mellitus without complications.
7. **S72.001A** – Fracture of the right femur, initial encounter.
8. **H25.813** – Bilateral age-related cataracts.
9. **L89.323** – Pressure ulcer of left heel, stage 3.
10. **S06.0X1A, W09.8XXA** – Concussion with loss of consciousness under 30 minutes (S06.0X1A) and fall from playground equipment (W09.8XXA), initial encounter.

INTERACTIVE CODING EXERCISES

Engaging in interactive coding exercises is a vital component of mastering ICD-10-CM coding. These exercises PROVIDE hands-on experience, allowing you to apply theoretical knowledge to practical scenarios. By working through real-world cases, you can enhance your problem-solving skills and ensure accurate code assignment. This section offers a series of carefully designed exercises aimed at reinforcing your understanding of coding principles and guidelines.

Basic Scenarios

Engaging with fundamental coding scenarios is essential for building a strong foundation in ICD-10-CM coding practices. These exercises provide practical experience, enabling coders to apply theoretical knowledge to real-world medical cases. The following scenarios are designed to enhance your understanding of accurate code assignment and reinforce key coding principles.

'Scenario 1: Routine Health Examination'

- **'Patient Details'**: 45-year-old male presenting for an annual physical examination.
- **'Medical History'**: No significant past medical history; non-smoker; moderate alcohol consumption.
- **'Examination Findings'**: Normal vital signs; unremarkable physical examination.
- **'Assessment'**: General adult medical examination without abnormal findings.
- 'ICD-10-CM **Code'**: Z00.00 – Encounter for general adult medical examination without abnormal findings.

'Scenario 2: Acute Upper Respiratory Infection'

- **'Patient Details'**: 30-year-old female presenting with a 3-day history of sore throat, cough, and nasal congestion.
- **'Medical History'**: No chronic illnesses; no known allergies.
- **'Examination Findings'**: Reddened pharynx; clear nasal discharge; lungs clear to auscultation.
- **'Assessment'**: Acute upper respiratory infection.
- 'ICD-10-CM **Code'**: J06.9 – Acute upper respiratory infection, unspecified.

'Scenario 3: Type 2 Diabetes Mellitus without Complications'

- **'Patient Details'**: 55-year-old male with a known history of type 2 diabetes mellitus.
- **'Medical History'**: Diagnosed 5 years ago; managed with oral hypoglycemic agents.
- **'Examination Findings'**: No signs of diabetic complications; recent HbA1c within target range.
- **'Assessment'**: Type 2 diabetes mellitus without complications.
- 'ICD-10-CM **Code'**: E11.9 – Type 2 diabetes mellitus without complications.

'Scenario 4: Essential (Primary) Hypertension'

- **'Patient Details'**: 60-year-old female presenting for routine follow-up of hypertension.
- **'Medical History'**: Hypertension diagnosed 10 years ago; controlled with medication.
- **'Examination Findings'**: Blood pressure: 130/80 mmHg; no signs of hypertensive complications.
- **'Assessment'**: Essential (primary) hypertension.
- **'ICD-10-CM Code'**: I10 – Essential (primary) hypertension.

'Scenario 5: Acute Cystitis without Hematuria'

- **'Patient Details'**: 28-year-old female presenting with dysuria and increased urinary frequency for 2 days.
- **'Medical History'**: No previous urinary tract infections; sexually active.
- **'Examination Findings'**: Suprapubic tenderness; urinalysis positive for leukocytes and nitrites.
- **'Assessment'**: Acute cystitis without hematuria.
- **'ICD-10-CM Code'**: N30.00 – Acute cystitis without hematuria.

'Scenario 6: Low Back Pain'

- **'Patient Details'**: 40-year-old male presenting with lower back pain for one week.
- **'Medical History'**: Works as a manual laborer; no history of trauma.
- **'Examination Findings'**: Tenderness over lumbar paraspinal muscles; limited range of motion due to pain.
- **'Assessment'**: Low back pain.
- **'ICD-10-CM Code'**: M54.5 – Low back pain.

'Scenario 7: Acute Pharyngitis'

- **'Patient Details'**: 22-year-old female presenting with a sore throat and fever for 2 days.
- **'Medical History'**: No significant past medical history; no known drug allergies.
- **'Examination Findings'**: Erythematous and swollen pharynx; no exudates; cervical lymphadenopathy present.
- **'Assessment'**: Acute pharyngitis.
- **'ICD-10-CM Code'**: J02.9 – Acute pharyngitis, unspecified.

'Scenario 8: Unspecified Abdominal Pain'

- **'Patient Details'**: 35-year-old male presenting with intermittent abdominal pain for 3 days.
- **'Medical History'**: No history of gastrointestinal disorders; no recent travel.
- **'Examination Findings'**: Mild diffuse abdominal tenderness; bowel sounds present; no rebound tenderness.
- **'Assessment'**: Unspecified abdominal pain.
- **'ICD-10-CM Code'**: R10.9 – Unspecified abdominal pain.

'Scenario 9: Allergic Rhinitis due to Pollen'

- **'Patient Details'**: 26-year-old female presenting with sneezing, nasal congestion, and itchy eyes during springtime.
- **'Medical History'**: Known seasonal allergies; no asthma.
- **'Examination Findings'**: Swollen nasal turbinates; clear nasal discharge; conjunctival injection.
- **'Assessment'**: Allergic rhinitis due to pollen.
- 'ICD-10-CM **Code'**: J30.1 – Allergic rhinitis due to pollen.

'Scenario 10: Obesity, Unspecified'

- **'Patient Details'**: 50-year-old male presenting for a wellness check
- **'Medical History'**: BMI not documented; no known comorbidities.
- **'Examination Findings'**: Weight above recommended range; no immediate complications.
- **'Assessment'**: Obesity, unspecified.
- 'ICD-10-CM **Code'**: E66.9 – Obesity, unspecified.

These basic scenarios provide practical coding exercises to reinforce your understanding of ICD-10-CM guidelines. By applying these concepts, you can enhance accuracy in medical documentation and coding assignments.

Introductory Exercises with Simple Cases

Practicing simple coding cases is essential for developing a strong foundation in ICD-10-CM coding. These exercises focus on straightforward medical conditions and commonly assigned codes, helping you build confidence and accuracy in code selection.

'Exercise 1: Routine Child Health Exam'

- **'Patient Details'**: 3-year-old male presenting for a routine pediatric wellness visit.
- **'Medical History'**: No chronic conditions; vaccinations up to date.
- **'Examination Findings'**: Normal growth and development; no abnormalities noted.
- **'Assessment'**: Routine child health check.
- 'ICD-10-CM **Code'**: Z00.129 – Encounter for routine child health examination without abnormal findings.

'Exercise 2: Acute Sinusitis'

- **'Patient Details'**: 32-year-old female with nasal congestion and facial pain for 10 days.
- **'Medical History'**: No prior sinus infections; no allergies.
- **'Examination Findings'**: Tenderness over maxillary sinuses; yellow nasal discharge.
- **'Assessment'**: Acute maxillary sinusitis.
- 'ICD-10-CM **Code'**: J01.00 – Acute maxillary sinusitis, unspecified.

'Exercise 3: Sprained Ankle'

- **'Patient Details'**: 27-year-old male who twisted his right ankle while jogging.
- **'Medical History'**: No previous ankle injuries.
- **'Examination Findings'**: Swelling and tenderness over the lateral ankle; no fractures on X-ray.
- **'Assessment'**: Sprain of right ankle.
- 'ICD-10-CM **Code'**: S93.401A – Sprain of unspecified ligament of right ankle, initial encounter.

'Exercise 4: Migraine without Aura'

- **'Patient Details'**: 45-year-old female with recurrent headaches, lasting several hours, accompanied by nausea and light sensitivity.
- **'Medical History'**: No aura; no known triggers.
- **'Examination Findings'**: Normal neurological exam.
- **'Assessment'**: Migraine without aura.
- **'ICD-10-CM Code'**: G43.909 – Migraine, unspecified, not intractable, without status migrainosus.

'Exercise 5: Otitis Media'

- **'Patient Details'**: 5-year-old male presenting with ear pain and fever for 3 days.
- **'Medical History'**: No prior ear infections.
- **'Examination Findings'**: Red, bulging tympanic membrane in the right ear.
- **'Assessment'**: Acute otitis media, right ear.
- **'ICD-10-CM Code'**: H66.91 – Otitis media, unspecified, right ear.

These introductory exercises help reinforce ICD-10-CM coding accuracy through simple, real-world cases. Practicing these cases ensures better understanding of medical terminology, documentation, and code selection.

Coding Drill: Assign the Correct ICD-10-CM Codes to 10 Brief Patient Scenarios

Review the patient scenarios below and assign the most accurate ICD-10-CM code for each case. This exercise helps strengthen your ability to quickly and accurately identify the correct diagnosis codes.

'Patient Scenarios'

1. 'A 50-year-old male presents for a follow-up visit for well-controlled type 2 diabetes mellitus with no complications.'
   ICD-10-CM **Code:** _____
2. 'A 7-year-old female is diagnosed with streptococcal pharyngitis after presenting with a sore throat and fever for two days.'
   ICD-10-CM **Code:** _____
3. 'A 30-year-old pregnant woman at 20 weeks gestation comes in for routine prenatal care. No complications noted.'
   ICD-10-CM **Code:** _____
4. 'A 42-year-old male presents with sudden-onset chest pain and is diagnosed with acute myocardial infarction of the left anterior descending artery.'
   ICD-10-CM **Code:** _____
5. 'A 60-year-old female is seen for chronic osteoarthritis in both knees, which causes pain and limited mobility.'
   ICD-10-CM **Code:** _____
6. 'A 28-year-old male presents after a motor vehicle accident with a confirmed concussion and loss of consciousness lasting 10 minutes.'
   ICD-10-CM **Code:** _____
7. 'A 5-year-old male is diagnosed with viral gastroenteritis after experiencing vomiting and diarrhea for two days.'
   ICD-10-CM **Code:** _____
8. 'A 35-year-old female with a known history of anxiety disorder is experiencing an acute anxiety episode.'
   ICD-10-CM **Code:** _____
9. 'A 48-year-old male is treated for a second-degree burn on his left forearm due to a cooking accident.'
   ICD-10-CM **Code:** _____
10. 'A 75-year-old female with osteoporosis is diagnosed with a vertebral compression fracture that occurred spontaneously.'
    ICD-10-CM **Code:** _____

Answer Key for Basic Scenarios:

1. **E11.9** – Type 2 diabetes mellitus without complications.
2. **J02.0** – Streptococcal pharyngitis.
3. **Z34.92** – Encounter for supervision of normal pregnancy, second trimester.
4. **I21.02** – ST-elevation (STEMI) myocardial infarction involving left anterior descending coronary artery.
5. **M17.0** – Bilateral primary osteoarthritis of knee.
6. **S06.0X1A** – Concussion with loss of consciousness of 10 minutes or less, initial encounter.
7. **A08.4** – Viral gastroenteritis, unspecified.
8. **F41.9** – Anxiety disorder, unspecified.
9. **T22.212A** – Second-degree burn of left forearm, initial encounter.
10. **M80.08XA** – Age-related osteoporosis with current pathological fracture of vertebra, initial encounter.

Intermediate Cases

Building upon foundational coding knowledge, intermediate cases present more complex scenarios that require a nuanced understanding of ICD-10-CM guidelines. These cases often involve multiple diagnoses, complications, or detailed medical histories, challenging coders to apply their skills in more intricate situations.

'Case 1: Postoperative Complications'

- **'Patient Details'**: 67-year-old female, status post total hip arthroplasty two weeks ago.
- **'Presenting Complaint'**: Increased pain and swelling in the operated hip.
- **'Examination Findings'**: Erythema, warmth, and tenderness over the surgical site; fever of 101.5°F.
- **'Assessment'**: Postoperative infection following hip replacement.
- **'ICD-10-CM Codes'**:
  - ○ T84.51XA – Infection and inflammatory reaction due to internal right hip prosthesis, initial encounter.
  - ○ Z96.641 – Presence of right artificial hip joint.

'Case 2: Diabetic Foot Ulcer with Peripheral Angiopathy'

- **'Patient Details'**: 58-year-old male with a 15-year history of type 2 diabetes mellitus.
- **'Presenting Complaint'**: Non-healing ulcer on the left foot.
- **'Examination Findings'**: Ulcer on the plantar surface of the left foot, measuring 2 cm in diameter; signs of peripheral arterial disease.
- **'Assessment'**: Diabetic foot ulcer with peripheral angiopathy.
- **'ICD-10-CM Codes'**:
  - ○ E11.621 – Type 2 diabetes mellitus with foot ulcer.
  - ○ L97.429 – Non-pressure chronic ulcer of left heel and midfoot with unspecified severity.
  - ○ I73.9 – Peripheral vascular disease, unspecified.

'Case 3: Acute Myocardial Infarction with Hypertension and Chronic Kidney Disease'

- **'Patient Details'**: 72-year-old male with a history of hypertension and stage 3 chronic kidney disease.
- **'Presenting Complaint'**: Severe chest pain radiating to the left arm.
- **'Examination Findings'**: Elevated blood pressure; ECG changes indicative of anterolateral wall myocardial infarction.
- **'Assessment'**: Acute ST-elevation myocardial infarction (STEMI) of the anterolateral wall.
- 'ICD-10-CM **Codes'**:
    - I21.09 – ST elevation (STEMI) myocardial infarction involving other coronary arteries of the anterior wall.
    - I12.9 – Hypertensive chronic kidney disease with stage 1 through stage 4 chronic kidney disease, or unspecified chronic kidney disease.
    - N18.3 – Chronic kidney disease, stage 3 (moderate).

'Case 4: Cerebrovascular Accident with Hemiplegia'

- **'Patient Details'**: 65-year-old female with atrial fibrillation.
- **'Presenting Complaint'**: Sudden onset of right-sided weakness and slurred speech.
- **'Examination Findings'**: Right-sided hemiplegia; CT scan confirms acute ischemic stroke in the left middle cerebral artery territory.
- **'Assessment**: Acute ischemic cerebrovascular accident with right-sided hemiplegia.
- 'ICD-10-CM **Codes'**:
    - I63.512 – Cerebral infarction due to unspecified occlusion or stenosis of left middle cerebral artery.
    - G81.91 – Hemiplegia, unspecified affecting right dominant side.
    - I48.91 – Unspecified atrial fibrillation.

'Case 5: Chronic Obstructive Pulmonary Disease with Acute Exacerbation and Pneumonia'

- **'Patient Details'**: 70-year-old male with a long-standing history of chronic obstructive pulmonary disease (COPD).
- **'Presenting Complaint'**: Increased shortness of breath, productive cough with purulent sputum, and fever.
- **'Examination Findings'**: Decreased breath sounds with wheezing; chest X-ray reveals right lower lobe pneumonia.
- **'Assessment**: Acute exacerbation of COPD with superimposed bacterial pneumonia.
- 'ICD-10-CM **Codes'**:
    - J44.0 – Chronic obstructive pulmonary disease with acute lower respiratory infection.
    - J18.1 – Lobar pneumonia, unspecified organism.
    - J44.1 – Chronic obstructive pulmonary disease with (acute) exacerbation.

'Case 6: Complicated Urinary Tract Infection in Pregnancy'

- **'Patient Details'**: 28-year-old pregnant female at 24 weeks gestation.
- **'Presenting Complaint'**: Dysuria, flank pain, and fever.
- **'Examination Findings'**: Costovertebral angle tenderness; urinalysis positive for nitrites and leukocyte esterase.
- **'Assessment'**: Acute pyelonephritis complicating pregnancy.
- 'ICD-10-CM **Codes'**:
    - O23.02 – Infections of kidney in pregnancy, second trimester.
    - N10 – Acute pyelonephritis.

○　Z3A.24 – 24 weeks gestation of pregnancy.

'Case 7: Rheumatoid Arthritis with Rheumatoid Lung Disease'

- **'Patient Details'**: 55-year-old female with a 10-year history of rheumatoid arthritis.
- **'Presenting Complaint'**: Chronic cough and dyspnea
- **'Examination Findings'**: Bilateral joint swelling and stiffness; chest X-ray shows interstitial lung disease.
- **'Assessment'**: Rheumatoid arthritis with associated rheumatoid lung disease.
- 'ICD-10-CM **Codes'**:
  - ○ M05.10 – Rheumatoid lung disease with rheumatoid arthritis, unspecified site.
  - ○ J84.10 – Unspecified interstitial pulmonary disease.

'Case 8: Open Fracture of the Tibia Due to Fall from Ladder'

- **'Patient Details'**: 43-year-old male fell from a ladder while painting his house.
- **'Presenting Complaint'**: Severe pain and visible deformity of the right leg.
- **'Examination Findings'**: Open fracture of the right tibia; X-ray confirms displaced fracture.
- **'Assessment'**: Open fracture of the right tibia due to fall from ladder.
- 'ICD-10-CM **Codes'**:
  - ○ S82.201B – Unspecified fracture of shaft of right tibia, initial encounter for open fracture type I or II.
  - ○ W11.XXXA – Fall from ladder, initial encounter.

'Case 9: Acute Appendicitis with Perforation'

- **'Patient Details'**: 28-year-old male with severe right lower quadrant pain and nausea for 24 hours.
- **'Presenting Complaint'**: Progressive abdominal pain with fever.
- **'Examination Findings'**: Guarding and rebound tenderness over McBurney's point; CT scan confirms perforated appendicitis.
- **'Assessment'**: Acute appendicitis with perforation.
- 'ICD-10-CM **Code'**:
  - ○ K35.32 – Acute appendicitis with perforation and localized peritonitis.

'Case 10: Gastroesophageal Reflux Disease with Esophagitis'

- **'Patient Details'**: 50-year-old male with a history of chronic acid reflux.
- **'Presenting Complaint'**: Burning sensation in chest, worse after meals and at night.
- **'Examination Findings'**: Endoscopy reveals erosive esophagitis.
- **'Assessment'**: Gastroesophageal reflux disease (GERD) with esophagitis.
- 'ICD-10-CM **Code'**:
  - ○ K21.0 – Gastroesophageal reflux disease with esophagitis.

Intermediate cases require a deeper understanding of ICD-10-CM guidelines, including sequencing, laterality, and complications. Practicing these scenarios helps coders refine their skills for handling real-world medical documentation challenges.

Clinical Scenarios of Medium Difficulty to Improve Decoding Skills

Medium-difficulty clinical scenarios require coders to interpret multiple conditions, complications, and coding conventions. These cases help refine coding accuracy by incorporating sequencing rules, laterality, and comorbid conditions.

'Scenario 1: Pneumonia with Chronic Heart Failure'

- **'Patient Details'**: 72-year-old male with a history of congestive heart failure (CHF).
- **'Presenting Complaint'**: Shortness of breath, productive cough, and fever for three days.
- **'Examination Findings'**: Crackles in both lung fields; chest X-ray confirms pneumonia.
- **'Assessment'**: Community-acquired pneumonia with chronic systolic heart failure.
- **'ICD-10-CM Codes'**:
  - 'J18.9 – Pneumonia, unspecified organism.'
  - 'I50.22 – Chronic systolic heart failure.'

'Scenario 2: Acute Diverticulitis with Rectal Bleeding'

- **'Patient Details'**: 60-year-old female with a history of diverticulosis.
- **'Presenting Complaint'**: Lower abdominal pain, fever, and bright red blood in stool.
- **'Examination Findings'**: Tenderness in the left lower quadrant; CT scan confirms acute diverticulitis with hemorrhage.
- **'Assessment'**: Acute diverticulitis of the large intestine with rectal bleeding.
- **'ICD-10-CM Code'**:
  - 'K57.33 – Diverticulitis of the large intestine with bleeding.'

'Scenario 3: Acute Deep Vein Thrombosis of Left Leg'

- **'Patient Details'**: 45-year-old male with a recent history of prolonged immobility due to surgery.
- **'Presenting Complaint'**: Swelling and pain in the left calf.
- **'Examination Findings'**: Ultrasound confirms acute deep vein thrombosis (DVT) in the left popliteal vein.
- **'Assessment'**: Acute DVT of the left lower extremity.
- **'ICD-10-CM Code'**:
  - 'I82.402 – Acute embolism and thrombosis of the left popliteal vein.'

'Scenario 4: Chronic Kidney Disease Stage 4 with Hypertension'

- **'Patient Details'**: 65-year-old female with long-standing hypertension and progressive renal decline.
- **'Presenting Complaint'**: Fatigue and swelling in lower extremities.
- **'Examination Findings'**: Elevated serum creatinine; eGFR indicates stage 4 chronic kidney disease (CKD).
- **'Assessment'**: Chronic kidney disease stage 4 with hypertensive nephropathy.
- **'ICD-10-CM Codes'**:
  - 'I12.9 – Hypertensive chronic kidney disease with stage 1-4 CKD.'
  - 'N18.4 – Chronic kidney disease, stage 4 (severe).'

'Scenario 5: Unstable Angina in a Patient with Hyperlipidemia'

- **'Patient Details'**: 55-year-old male with hyperlipidemia and family history of heart disease.
- **'Presenting Complaint'**: Chest pain at rest and with exertion.
- **'Examination Findings'**: ECG shows ischemic changes; cardiac enzymes normal.
- **'Assessment'**: Unstable angina with hyperlipidemia.
- **'ICD-10-CM Codes'**:
  - 'I20.0 – Unstable angina.'
  - 'E78.5 – Hyperlipidemia, unspecified.'

'Scenario 6: Complicated Urinary Tract Infection Due to E. Coli'

- **'Patient Details'**: 40-year-old female with recurrent urinary tract infections (UTIs).
- **'Presenting Complaint'**: Dysuria, urgency, and fever for two days.
- **'Examination Findings'**: Urine culture positive for Escherichia coli (E. coli).
- **'Assessment'**: Complicated UTI caused by E. coli.
- **'ICD-10-CM Codes'**:
  - 'N39.0 – Urinary tract infection, site not specified.'
  - 'B96.20 – Unspecified Escherichia coli as the cause of disease.'

'Scenario 7: Acute Pancreatitis with Alcohol Dependence'

- **'Patient Details'**: 50-year-old male with chronic alcohol use.
- **'Presenting Complaint'**: Severe upper abdominal pain radiating to the back, nausea, and vomiting.
- **'Examination Findings'**: Elevated amylase and lipase levels; imaging confirms acute pancreatitis.
- **'Assessment'**: Acute pancreatitis due to chronic alcohol use.
- **'ICD-10-CM Codes'**:
  - 'K85.20 – Alcohol-induced acute pancreatitis without necrosis or infection.'
  - 'F10.20 – Alcohol dependence, uncomplicated.'

'Scenario 8: Traumatic Brain Injury with Loss of Consciousness'

- **'Patient Details'**: 30-year-old female involved in a motor vehicle accident.
- **'Presenting Complaint'**: Headache, dizziness, and memory loss.
- **'Examination Findings'**: CT scan reveals mild traumatic brain injury with loss of consciousness for 15 minutes.
- **'Assessment'**: Concussion with brief loss of consciousness.
- **'ICD-10-CM Code'**:
  - 'S06.0X1A – Concussion with loss of consciousness of 30 minutes or less, initial encounter.'

'Scenario 9: Right Rotator Cuff Tear with Shoulder Pain'

- **'Patient Details'**: 60-year-old male with worsening shoulder pain for six months.
- **'Presenting Complaint'**: Difficulty lifting arm and performing daily tasks.
- **'Examination Findings'**: MRI confirms full-thickness tear of the right rotator cuff.
- **'Assessment'**: Right rotator cuff tear with shoulder pain.
- 'ICD-10-CM **Codes**':
    - 'M75.121 – Complete rotator cuff tear or rupture of right shoulder, not specified as traumatic.'
    - 'M25.511 – Pain in right shoulder.'

'Scenario 10: Gastrointestinal Bleeding Due to Gastric Ulcer'

- **'Patient Details'**: 48-year-old female with a history of NSAID use.
- **'Presenting Complaint'**: Dark stools and mild abdominal discomfort.
- **'Examination Findings'**: Endoscopy reveals a bleeding gastric ulcer.
- **'Assessment'**: Gastric ulcer with gastrointestinal hemorrhage.
- 'ICD-10-CM **Code**':
    - 'K25.4 – Gastric ulcer with hemorrhage.'

Medium-difficulty clinical cases challenge coders to analyze multiple diagnoses, complications, and underlying conditions. These exercises improve accuracy in applying ICD-10-CM guidelines while reinforcing real-world medical coding skills.

Case-Based Exercise: Analyze 7 Detailed Cases and Select the Correct Codes

Read each case carefully and assign the correct ICD-10-CM code(s) based on the details provided. Consider sequencing, laterality, and complications when selecting the appropriate codes.

'Case 1: Hypertension with Chronic Kidney Disease'

- **'Patient Details'**: 70-year-old male with a history of hypertension and stage 3 chronic kidney disease (CKD).
- **'Presenting Complaint'**: Fatigue and mild lower extremity swelling.
- **'Examination Findings'**: Blood pressure 150/95 mmHg; labs show decreased glomerular filtration rate.
- **'Assessment'**: Hypertensive chronic kidney disease, stage 3.
- 'ICD-10-CM **Codes**': _____

'Case 2: Acute Stroke with Left-Sided Weakness'

- **'Patient Details'**: 68-year-old female with history of atrial fibrillation.
- **'Presenting Complaint'**: Sudden onset of slurred speech and weakness in the left arm and leg.
- **'Examination Findings'**: CT confirms acute ischemic stroke in the right middle cerebral artery.
- **'Assessment'**: Acute ischemic stroke with left-sided hemiparesis.
- 'ICD-10-CM **Codes**': _____

'Case 3: Type 2 Diabetes with Neuropathy'

- **'Patient Details'**: 55-year-old male with a 10-year history of type 2 diabetes mellitus.
- **'Presenting Complaint'**: Numbness and tingling in both feet.
- **'Examination Findings'**: Loss of sensation in bilateral lower extremities; HbA1c elevated.
- **'Assessment'**: Type 2 diabetes with diabetic neuropathy.
- 'ICD-10-CM **Codes'**: _____

'Case 4: Fractured Wrist Due to Fall'

- **'Patient Details'**: 45-year-old female tripped and landed on her outstretched right hand.
- **'Presenting Complaint'**: Severe wrist pain and swelling.
- **'Examination Findings'**: X-ray confirms displaced distal radius fracture.
- **'Assessment'**: Closed displaced fracture of the right distal radius due to a fall.
- 'ICD-10-CM **Codes'**: _____

'Case 5: COPD with Acute Exacerbation'

- **'Patient Details'**: 72-year-old male with a history of chronic obstructive pulmonary disease (COPD).
- **'Presenting Complaint'**: Worsening shortness of breath and increased sputum production.
- **'Examination Findings'**: Decreased breath sounds; chest X-ray shows hyperinflation.
- **'Assessment'**: COPD with acute exacerbation.
- 'ICD-10-CM **Codes'**: _____

'Case 6: Gastrointestinal Bleeding with Anemia'

- **'Patient Details'**: 60-year-old female with a history of peptic ulcer disease.
- **'Presenting Complaint'**: Fatigue and dark stools for one week.
- **'Examination Findings'**: Endoscopy confirms bleeding gastric ulcer; hemoglobin low.
- **'Assessment'**: Gastrointestinal bleeding with iron deficiency anemia due to chronic blood loss.
- 'ICD-10-CM **Codes'**: _____

'Case 7: Right Shoulder Pain Due to Rotator Cuff Tear'

- **'Patient Details'**: 50-year-old male with chronic right shoulder pain after a sports injury.
- **'Presenting Complaint'**: Difficulty lifting arm above shoulder level.
- **'Examination Findings'**: MRI confirms a full-thickness tear of the right supraspinatus tendon.
- **'Assessment'**: Right rotator cuff tear.
- 'ICD-10-CM **Codes'**: _____

Answer Key for Intermediate Cases

Case 1: Hypertension with Chronic Kidney Disease

- **I12.9** – Hypertensive chronic kidney disease with stage 1 through stage 4 CKD, or unspecified CKD
- **N18.3** – Chronic kidney disease, stage 3

Case 2: Acute Stroke with Left-Sided Weakness

- **I63.511** – Cerebral infarction due to occlusion or stenosis of right middle cerebral artery
- **G81.94** – Hemiplegia, affecting left nondominant side
- **I48.91** – Unspecified atrial fibrillation (if still present)

Case 3: Type 2 Diabetes with Neuropathy

- **E11.40** – Type 2 diabetes mellitus with diabetic neuropathy, unspecified

Case 4: Fractured Wrist Due to Fall

- **S52.501A** – Displaced fracture of distal end of right radius, initial encounter for closed fracture
- **W19.XXXA** – Unspecified fall, initial encounter

Case 5: COPD with Acute Exacerbation

- **J44.1** – Chronic obstructive pulmonary disease with (acute) exacerbation

Case 6: Gastrointestinal Bleeding with Anemia

- **K25.4** – Chronic gastric ulcer with hemorrhage
- **D50.0** – Iron deficiency anemia secondary to blood loss (chronic)

Case 7: Right Shoulder Pain Due to Rotator Cuff Tear

- **M75.121** – Complete rotator cuff tear or rupture of right shoulder, not specified as traumatic

By ensuring accurate ICD-10-CM coding, healthcare professionals can improve documentation, facilitate reimbursement, and enhance patient care.

Advanced Real-World Cases

Engaging with advanced real-world cases enhances proficiency in ICD-10-CM coding by challenging coders to navigate complex medical scenarios. These cases often involve multiple comorbidities, complications, and require a deep understanding of coding conventions and guidelines.

'Case 1: Drug-Induced Cataracts Due to Long-Term Glucocorticoid Use'

- **Patient Details**: 72-year-old male on long-term glucocorticoid therapy for chronic inflammatory condition.
- **Presenting Complaint**: Progressive bilateral vision blurriness.
- **Examination Findings**: Ophthalmologic assessment reveals bilateral cataracts.
- **Assessment**: Bilateral drug-induced cataracts secondary to prolonged glucocorticoid use.
- ICD-10-CM **Codes**:
    - H26.33 – Drug-induced cataract, bilateral.
    - T38.0X5A – Adverse effect of glucocorticoids and synthetic analogues, initial encounter.

'Case 2: COVID-19 Presenting with Acute Atopic Conjunctivitis'

- **Patient Details**: 45-year-old female with recent exposure to a COVID-19 positive individual.
- **Presenting Complaint**: Red, itchy, sticky right eye; mild fever; lethargy.
- **Examination Findings**: Atopic conjunctivitis in the right eye; mild wheezing noted upon chest examination.
- **Assessment**: Acute atopic conjunctivitis associated with confirmed COVID-19 infection.
- ICD-10-CM **Codes**:
    - U07.1 – COVID-19.
    - H10.11 – Acute atopic conjunctivitis, right eye.

'Case 3: Acute Myocardial Infarction with Subsequent Cerebrovascular Accident'

- **Patient Details**: 68-year-old male with a history of hypertension and hyperlipidemia.
- **Presenting Complaint**: Severe chest pain radiating to the left arm, followed by sudden onset of right-sided weakness and speech difficulties.
- **Examination Findings**: ECG indicates ST-elevation myocardial infarction (STEMI); CT scan reveals acute ischemic stroke in the left middle cerebral artery territory.
- **Assessment**: Acute STEMI complicated by subsequent cerebrovascular accident (stroke).
- ICD-10-CM **Codes**:
    - I21.3 – ST elevation (STEMI) myocardial infarction of unspecified site.
    - I63.512 – Cerebral infarction due to unspecified occlusion or stenosis of left middle cerebral artery.

'Case 4: Severe Sepsis Due to Pneumonia with Acute Respiratory Failure'

- **Patient Details**: 75-year-old female with a history of chronic obstructive pulmonary disease (COPD).
- **Presenting Complaint**: Shortness of breath, high fever, and productive cough.
- **Examination Findings**: Chest X-ray shows lobar pneumonia; arterial blood gases indicate acute hypoxemic respiratory failure; blood cultures positive for Streptococcus pneumoniae.
- **Assessment**: Severe sepsis secondary to pneumococcal pneumonia with acute respiratory failure.
- ICD-10-CM **Codes**:
    - A40.3 – Sepsis due to Streptococcus pneumoniae.

- J13 – Pneumonia due to Streptococcus pneumoniae.
- R65.20 – Severe sepsis without septic shock.
- J96.00 – Acute respiratory failure, unspecified whether with hypoxia or hypercapnia.

'Case 5: Complicated Type 2 Diabetes Mellitus with Diabetic Nephropathy and Hypertensive Chronic Kidney Disease'

- **Patient Details**: 60-year-old male with a long-standing history of type 2 diabetes mellitus and hypertension.
- **Presenting Complaint**: Persistent proteinuria and elevated serum creatinine levels.
- **Examination Findings**: Signs of chronic kidney disease; blood pressure consistently elevated despite medication adherence.
- **Assessment**: Diabetic nephropathy with concurrent hypertensive chronic kidney disease, stage 3.
- ICD-10-CM **Codes**:
  - E11.22 – Type 2 diabetes mellitus with diabetic chronic kidney disease.
  - I12.9 – Hypertensive chronic kidney disease with stage 1 through stage 4 chronic kidney disease, or unspecified chronic kidney disease.
  - N18.3 – Chronic kidney disease, stage 3 (moderate).

'Case 6: Traumatic Brain Injury with Prolonged Loss of Consciousness'

- **Patient Details**: 30-year-old male involved in a high-speed motor vehicle collision.
- **Presenting Complaint**: Unresponsive at the scene; regained consciousness after approximately 24 hours.
- **Examination Findings**: CT scan reveals diffuse axonal injury; Glasgow Coma Scale score of 10 upon admission.
- **Assessment**: Severe traumatic brain injury with prolonged loss of consciousness.
- ICD-10-CM **Codes**:
  - S06.2X5A – Diffuse traumatic brain injury with loss of consciousness of 6 hours to 24 hours, initial encounter.
  - R40.2311 – Glasgow coma scale score 9-12, initial encounter.

'Case 7: Postoperative Deep Vein Thrombosis Following Hip Replacement Surgery'

- **Patient Details**: 65-year-old female, two weeks post right total hip arthroplasty.
- **Presenting Complaint**: Swelling and pain in the right leg.
- **Examination Findings**: Doppler ultrasound confirms deep vein thrombosis (DVT) in the right femoral vein.
- **Assessment**: Postoperative deep vein thrombosis following hip replacement surgery.
- ICD-10-CM **Codes**:
  - I82.401 – Acute embolism and thrombosis of unspecified deep veins of right lower extremity.
  - T81.72XA – Complication of a surgical procedure, deep vein thrombosis, initial encounter.
  - Z96.641 – Presence of right artificial hip joint.

'Case 8: Severe Burn Injuries Due to House Fire'

- **Patient Details**: 42-year-old male rescued from a house fire.
- **Presenting Complaint**: Burns on the face, chest, and both arms.
- **Examination Findings**: Second-degree burns on the chest and arms; third-degree burns on the face; inhalation injury suspected.
- **Assessment**: Severe burns involving multiple body regions with suspected smoke inhalation injury.
- ICD-10-CM **Codes**:
    - T21.21XA – Second-degree burn of chest wall, initial encounter.
    - T22.299A – Second-degree burn of multiple sites of upper limb, initial encounter.
    - T20.30XA – Third-degree burn of face, unspecified site, initial encounter.
    - T59.81XA – Toxic effect of smoke, initial encounter.

'Case 9: Multiple Fractures from a High-Impact Fall'

- **Patient Details**: 35-year-old female who fell from a third-story balcony.
- **Presenting Complaint**: Severe pain in left leg, right arm, and ribs.
- **Examination Findings**: X-rays confirm a closed left femoral shaft fracture, a closed right humerus fracture, and multiple rib fractures.
- **Assessment**: Multiple traumatic fractures from a high-impact fall.
- ICD-10-CM **Codes**:
    - S72.302A – Unspecified fracture of shaft of left femur, initial encounter.
    - S42.301A – Unspecified fracture of shaft of right humerus, initial encounter.
    - S22.41XA – Multiple rib fractures, initial encounter.
    - W13.2XXA – Fall from, out of, or through a balcony, initial encounter.

'Case 10: HIV Disease with Kaposi Sarcoma'

- **Patient Details**: 50-year-old male with a known history of HIV infection.
- **Presenting Complaint**: Multiple reddish-purple skin lesions appearing on the lower extremities.
- **Examination Findings**: Biopsy confirms Kaposi sarcoma.
- **Assessment**: HIV disease with Kaposi sarcoma.
- ICD-10-CM **Codes**:
    - B20 – Human immunodeficiency virus (HIV) disease.
    - C46.0 – Kaposi sarcoma of skin.

Advanced real-world cases require coders to apply a deep understanding of ICD-10-CM coding rules, including sequencing, complications, and comorbid conditions. Mastering these cases enhances accuracy in coding complex medical scenarios, ensuring compliance and proper reimbursement.

Complex Clinical Cases to Test Advanced Skills

Complex medical cases require coders to apply ICD-10-CM guidelines with precision, considering multiple diagnoses, complications, and underlying conditions. These cases test advanced coding skills, requiring proper sequencing and attention to official coding conventions.

Case 1: Multisystem Organ Failure Due to Septic Shock

- **Patient Details**: 67-year-old male with a history of diabetes and chronic kidney disease.
- **Presenting Complaint**: High fever, confusion, and low blood pressure.
- **Examination Findings**: Blood cultures positive for E. coli; lactic acidosis; acute respiratory failure; elevated creatinine levels indicating worsening kidney function.
- **Assessment**: Sepsis due to E. coli with septic shock, multisystem organ failure involving acute kidney and respiratory failure.
- ICD-10-CM **Codes**:
    - A41.51 – Sepsis due to Escherichia coli.
    - R65.21 – Severe sepsis with septic shock.
    - J96.00 – Acute respiratory failure, unspecified.
    - N17.9 – Acute kidney failure, unspecified.

Case 2: Acute Stroke with Hemorrhagic Transformation and Dysphagia

- **Patient Details**: 74-year-old female with a history of hypertension and atrial fibrillation.
- **Presenting Complaint**: Left-sided weakness and difficulty speaking.
- **Examination Findings**: CT confirms an acute ischemic stroke in the right middle cerebral artery with hemorrhagic transformation. Swallow study reveals dysphagia.
- **Assessment**: Ischemic stroke with hemorrhagic conversion, dysphagia.
- ICD-10-CM **Codes**:
    - I63.50 – Cerebral infarction due to unspecified occlusion or stenosis of unspecified cerebral artery.
    - I61.9 – Nontraumatic intracerebral hemorrhage, unspecified.
    - R13.10 – Dysphagia, unspecified.

Case 3: Metastatic Lung Cancer with Pathologic Vertebral Fracture

- **Patient Details**: 60-year-old male with a known history of stage IV lung cancer.
- **Presenting Complaint**: Severe back pain and progressive weakness in lower extremities.
- **Examination Findings**: MRI confirms vertebral compression fractures due to bone metastases.
- **Assessment**: Metastatic non-small cell lung cancer to bone with pathologic vertebral fractures.
- ICD-10-CM **Codes**:
    - C34.90 – Malignant neoplasm of unspecified part of unspecified bronchus or lung.
    - C79.51 – Secondary malignant neoplasm of bone.
    - M84.58XA – Pathological fracture in neoplastic disease, other specified site, initial encounter.

Case 4: Complicated Pregnancy with Gestational Diabetes and Preeclampsia

- **Patient Details**: 32-year-old female at 30 weeks gestation.
- **Presenting Complaint**: Elevated blood pressure, proteinuria, and abnormal glucose levels.
- **Examination Findings**: Gestational diabetes confirmed via glucose tolerance test; elevated blood pressure with proteinuria.
- **Assessment**: Gestational diabetes with preeclampsia in the third trimester.
- ICD-10-CM **Codes**:
    - O24.419 – Gestational diabetes mellitus in pregnancy, unspecified control.
    - O14.03 – Severe preeclampsia, third trimester.
    - Z3A.30 – 30 weeks gestation of pregnancy.

Case 5: Traumatic Brain Injury with Subdural Hematoma and Coma

- **Patient Details**: 29-year-old male involved in a high-speed car accident.
- **Presenting Complaint**: Unconscious at the scene with a Glasgow Coma Scale (GCS) of 6.
- **Examination Findings**: CT scan reveals a large subdural hematoma with midline shift; intubated and placed on mechanical ventilation.
- **Assessment**: Severe traumatic brain injury with subdural hematoma and coma.
- ICD-10-CM **Codes**:
    - S06.5X5A – Traumatic subdural hemorrhage with loss of consciousness greater than 24 hours, initial encounter.

Case 6: Acute Respiratory Distress Syndrome with COVID-19 and Pneumonia

- **Patient Details**: 55-year-old male with obesity and hypertension.
- **Presenting Complaint**: Severe shortness of breath, fever, and hypoxia.
- **Examination Findings**: Chest X-ray shows bilateral infiltrates; RT-PCR confirms COVID-19; intubated due to worsening respiratory distress.
- **Assessment**: COVID-19 pneumonia with acute respiratory distress syndrome (ARDS).
- ICD-10-CM **Codes**:
    - U07.1 – COVID-19.
    - J12.82 – Pneumonia due to COVID-19.
    - J80 – Acute respiratory distress syndrome.

Case 7: End-Stage Liver Disease with Hepatorenal Syndrome

- **Patient Details**: 58-year-old female with cirrhosis due to chronic hepatitis C.
- **Presenting Complaint**: Worsening ascites, confusion, and oliguria.
- **Examination Findings**: Elevated bilirubin, creatinine, and ammonia levels; paracentesis performed for severe ascites.
- **Assessment**: End-stage liver disease with hepatorenal syndrome.
- ICD-10-CM **Codes**:
    - K74.60 – Hepatic fibrosis with cirrhosis, unspecified.
    - N25.81 – Hepatorenal syndrome.
    - B18.2 – Chronic viral hepatitis C.

Case 8: Necrotizing Fasciitis with Sepsis and Septic Shock

- **Patient Details**: 50-year-old male with poorly controlled diabetes mellitus.
- **Presenting Complaint**: Rapidly worsening pain, redness, and swelling in the right lower leg.
- **Examination Findings**: Crepitus and skin necrosis noted; blood cultures positive for Group A Streptococcus; patient is hypotensive and requires vasopressors.
- **Assessment**: Necrotizing fasciitis with sepsis and septic shock.
- ICD-10-CM **Codes**:
  - M72.6 – Necrotizing fasciitis.
  - A41.81 – Sepsis due to Group A Streptococcus.
  - R65.21 – Severe sepsis with septic shock.

Case 9: Spinal Cord Injury with Quadriplegia

- **Patient Details**: 38-year-old male who sustained a cervical spinal cord injury after diving into shallow water.
- **Presenting Complaint**: Complete loss of motor and sensory function below the neck.
- **Examination Findings**: MRI confirms C4-C5 spinal cord injury with complete loss of function.
- **Assessment**: Complete quadriplegia due to spinal cord injury.
- ICD-10-CM **Codes**:
  - S14.109A – Complete lesion of unspecified level of cervical spinal cord, initial encounter.
  - S14.101A – Complete lesion of C1-C4 level of cervical spinal cord, initial encounter, to accurately reflect the injury.

Case 10: Post-Transplant Rejection of Kidney Graft

- **Patient Details**: 49-year-old female with a history of renal transplant one year ago.
- **Presenting Complaint**: Increased creatinine levels and reduced urine output.
- **Examination Findings**: Renal biopsy confirms acute kidney transplant rejection.
- **Assessment**: Acute kidney transplant rejection.
- ICD-10-CM **Codes**:
  - T86.13 – Kidney transplant rejection.
  - Z94.0 – Kidney transplant status.

Complex clinical cases require advanced critical thinking, precise sequencing, and an in-depth understanding of ICD-10-CM guidelines. Mastering these scenarios prepares coders for high-level medical documentation and real-world healthcare challenges.

Challenge Yourself: Decode Multi-Layered Cases with Comorbidities and Unusual Presentations

Multi-layered cases often involve multiple comorbidities, rare conditions, and complex clinical presentations. These scenarios challenge coders to apply advanced ICD-10-CM coding skills, ensuring proper sequencing, specificity, and adherence to official guidelines.

Case 1: Acute Coronary Syndrome with Shock Liver and Atrial Fibrillation

- **Patient Details**: 68-year-old male with a history of hypertension and atrial fibrillation.
- **Presenting Complaint**: Severe chest pain, nausea, and dizziness.
- **Examination Findings**: Elevated troponins; ECG shows ST depression; echocardiogram reveals left ventricular dysfunction. Liver enzymes significantly elevated, indicating ischemic hepatitis (shock liver).
- **Assessment**: Acute coronary syndrome with ischemic hepatitis and underlying atrial fibrillation.
- ICD-10-CM **Codes**:
    - I24.9 – Acute ischemic heart disease, unspecified.
    - K72.00 – Acute and subacute hepatic failure without coma.
    - I48.91 – Unspecified atrial fibrillation.

Case 2: Autoimmune Hemolytic Anemia with Systemic Lupus Erythematosus

- **Patient Details**: 45-year-old female with a known history of **systemic lupus erythematosus (SLE).**
- **Presenting Complaint**: Severe fatigue, jaundice, and pallor.
- **Examination Findings**: Low hemoglobin, elevated bilirubin, and a positive Coombs test confirming autoimmune hemolytic anemia.
- **Assessment**: Autoimmune hemolytic anemia secondary to systemic lupus erythematosus.
- ICD-10-CM **Codes**:
    - D59.0 – Autoimmune hemolytic anemia.
    - M32.10 – Systemic lupus erythematosus, organ or system involvement unspecified.

Case 3: COVID-19 with Guillain-Barré Syndrome and Acute Respiratory Failure

- **Patient Details**: 55-year-old male with no significant past medical history.
- **Presenting Complaint**: Progressive weakness, difficulty breathing, and tingling in the extremities.
- **Examination Findings**: Confirmed COVID-19 infection, ascending muscle paralysis, and reduced reflexes. Required mechanical ventilation due to acute respiratory failure.
- **Assessment**: COVID-19 associated Guillain-Barré syndrome with acute respiratory failure.
- ICD-10-CM **Codes**:
    - U07.1 – COVID-19.
    - G61.0 – Guillain-Barré syndrome.
    - J96.00 – Acute respiratory failure, unspecified.

Case 4: Malignant Hypertension with Acute Kidney Injury and Hypertensive Encephalopathy

- **Patient Details**: 50-year-old male with a long history of poorly controlled hypertension.
- **Presenting Complaint**: Sudden confusion, blurry vision, and severe headache.
- **Examination Findings**: Blood pressure 230/130 mmHg; creatinine elevated; altered mental status. Diagnosed with hypertensive emergency leading to acute kidney injury and hypertensive encephalopathy.
- **Assessment**: Malignant hypertension with acute kidney injury and encephalopathy.
- ICD-10-CM **Codes**:
    - I67.4 – Hypertensive encephalopathy.
    - I12.9 – Hypertensive chronic kidney disease, stage 1-4 or unspecified.
    - N17.9 – Acute kidney failure, unspecified.

Case 5: Type 1 Diabetes with Diabetic Ketoacidosis and Gastroparesis

- **Patient Details**: 30-year-old female with type 1 diabetes mellitus since childhood.
- **Presenting Complaint**: Nausea, vomiting, and severe abdominal pain for two days.
- **Examination Findings**: Blood glucose >400 mg/dL, arterial blood gas shows metabolic acidosis, ketones present in urine. Gastric emptying study confirms gastroparesis due to diabetes.
- **Assessment**: Type 1 diabetes mellitus with diabetic ketoacidosis (DKA) and diabetic gastroparesis.
- ICD-10-CM **Codes**:
    - E10.10 – Type 1 diabetes mellitus with ketoacidosis without coma.
    - E10.43 – Type 1 diabetes mellitus with diabetic autonomic (gastroparesis) neuropathy.

Case 6: End-Stage Renal Disease with Hyperparathyroidism and Bone Fracture

- **Patient Details**: 65-year-old male on hemodialysis for end-stage renal disease (ESRD).
- **Presenting Complaint**: Severe bone pain and recent fall.
- **Examination Findings**: X-ray confirms pathologic femur fracture; blood work shows secondary hyperparathyroidism due to chronic kidney disease.
- **Assessment**: End-stage renal disease with secondary hyperparathyroidism and pathologic femur fracture.
- ICD-10-CM **Codes**:
    - N18.6 – End-stage renal disease.
    - N25.81 – Secondary hyperparathyroidism of renal origin.
    - M84.40XA – Pathologic fracture, unspecified site, initial encounter.

Case 7: Metastatic Breast Cancer with Paraneoplastic Syndrome and Hypercalcemia

- **Patient Details**: 55-year-old female with stage IV breast cancer.
- **Presenting Complaint**: Fatigue, confusion, and severe muscle weakness.
- **Examination Findings**: Calcium levels >13 mg/dL; PET scan confirms bone metastases. Diagnosed with paraneoplastic hypercalcemia due to metastatic breast cancer.
- **Assessment**: Metastatic breast cancer with hypercalcemia due to paraneoplastic syndrome.
- ICD-10-CM **Codes**:
    - C50.919 – Malignant neoplasm of unspecified breast, female.
    - C79.51 – Secondary malignant neoplasm of bone.
    - E83.52 – Hypercalcemia.

Case 8: Spontaneous Pneumothorax in a Patient with Marfan Syndrome

- **Patient Details**: 29-year-old male with a known history of Marfan syndrome.
- **Presenting Complaint**: Sudden-onset sharp chest pain and shortness of breath.
- **Examination Findings**: Chest X-ray confirms spontaneous pneumothorax. No history of trauma or lung disease.
- **Assessment**: Primary spontaneous pneumothorax due to Marfan syndrome.
- ICD-10-CM **Codes**:
    - J93.11 – Primary spontaneous pneumothorax.
    - Q87.40 – Marfan syndrome.

Case 9: Parkinson's Disease with Dementia and Frequent Falls

- **Patient Details**: 76-year-old male with a history of Parkinson's disease.
- **Presenting Complaint**: Progressive memory loss, recurrent falls, and worsening tremors.
- **Examination Findings**: Neurological exam shows bradykinesia, resting tremor, and postural instability. Mini-Mental State Examination (MMSE) indicates moderate dementia.
- **Assessment**: Parkinson's disease with dementia and frequent falls.
- ICD-10-CM **Codes**:
    - G20 – Parkinson's disease.
    - G31.83 – Dementia with Lewy bodies.
    - R29.6 – Repeated falls.

Case 10: Necrotizing Pancreatitis with Multiple Organ Failure

- **Patient Details**: 58-year-old male with a history of **chronic alcohol abuse.**
- **Presenting Complaint**: Severe epigastric pain, nausea, and vomiting.
- **Examination Findings**: CT scan confirms necrotizing pancreatitis; patient develops acute kidney and respiratory failure.
- **Assessment**: Acute necrotizing pancreatitis with multiple organ failure.
- ICD-10-CM **Codes**:
    - K85.8 – Other acute pancreatitis.
    - N17.9 – Acute kidney failure, unspecified.
    - J96.00 – Acute respiratory failure, unspecified.

These **multi-layered cases** challenge coders to think critically and apply **advanced** ICD-10-CM coding principles. Success in coding these cases requires a deep understanding of **comorbidities, complications, and sequencing rules** to ensure accuracy and compliance.

SPECIALTY CODING SECTIONS

Specialty coding involves the application of ICD-10-CM codes tailored to specific medical fields, ensuring precise documentation and optimal reimbursement. Each specialty encounters unique conditions and procedures, necessitating a thorough understanding of the latest coding updates and guidelines pertinent to their practice area. Staying informed about these specialty-specific codes is crucial for accurate reporting and compliance in today's dynamic healthcare environment.

Inpatient vs. Outpatient Coding

Documentation and Coding Practices

- **Inpatient Coding**:
    - Coders assign codes for all diagnoses, including unconfirmed or suspected conditions, as documented at the time of discharge.
    - Utilizes ICD-10-CM for diagnoses and ICD-10-PCS for procedures.
    - Requires detailed documentation of the patient's entire hospital stay, including daily progress notes, operative reports, and discharge summaries.
- **Outpatient Coding**:
    - Codes are assigned only for confirmed diagnoses; if a definitive diagnosis is not available, symptoms and signs are coded.
    - Employs ICD-10-CM for diagnoses and CPT/HCPCS for procedures and services.
    - Documentation focuses on individual encounters, such as physician office visits or same-day surgeries, emphasizing the specific services provided during each visit.

Payment Systems

- **Inpatient Coding**:
    - Operates under the Inpatient Prospective Payment System (IPPS).
    - Patients are classified into Diagnosis-Related Groups (DRGs), which determine reimbursement rates based on the patient's diagnoses and procedures.
- **Outpatient Coding**:
    - Utilizes the Outpatient Prospective Payment System (OPPS).
    - Services are categorized into Ambulatory Payment Classifications (APCs), with reimbursement based on the specific procedures and services rendered.

Code Sets and Guidelines

- **Inpatient Coding**:
    - Uses ICD-10-CM for reporting diagnoses and ICD-10-PCS for inpatient procedures.
    - Follows guidelines set forth by the Centers for Medicare & Medicaid Services (CMS) and the ICD-10-CM Official Guidelines for Coding and Reporting.
- **Outpatient Coding**:
    - Employs ICD-10-CM for diagnoses and Current Procedural Terminology (CPT) along with Healthcare Common Procedure Coding System (HCPCS) for procedures and services.
    - Adheres to guidelines from the American Medical Association (AMA) for CPT and CMS for HCPCS codes.

Recent Updates

- **Evaluation and Management (E/M) Services**:
  - As of January 1, 2024, significant updates have been made to E/M coding guidelines affecting both inpatient and outpatient settings.
  - Providers can now select E/M service levels based on either Medical Decision Making (MDM) or total time spent on the date of the encounter.
  - The definition of "per day" has been clarified to mean that multiple visits on the same calendar date in the same setting should be reported as a single service.

- **Prolonged Services**:
  - New codes have been introduced for reporting prolonged services beyond the typical time associated with primary E/M services.
  - These codes account for the additional time and complexity involved in patient care, applicable in both inpatient and outpatient settings.

Understanding these aspects of inpatient and outpatient coding is essential for accurate documentation, compliance, and optimal reimbursement in healthcare settings.

Key Differences between Inpatient and Outpatient Coding with Practical Examples

Coding Systems

- **Inpatient Coding**:
  - Utilizes ICD-10-CM for diagnoses and **ICD-10-PCS** for procedures.
  - *Example*: A patient admitted for coronary artery bypass surgery would have diagnoses coded with ICD-10-CM and the surgical procedure coded with ICD-10-PCS.
- **Outpatient Coding**:
  - Employs ICD-10-CM for diagnoses and **CPT/HCPCS** for procedures.
  - *Example*: A patient visiting a clinic for a mole removal would have the diagnosis coded with ICD-10-CM and the procedure coded with a CPT code.

Length of Stay

- **Inpatient Coding**:
  - Applies to patients formally admitted to a healthcare facility, typically involving stays longer than 24 hours.
  - *Example*: A patient admitted for pneumonia treatment over several days would be considered inpatient.
- **Outpatient Coding**:
  - Pertains to services where patients receive care without formal admission, usually less than 24 hours.
  - *Example*: A patient receiving same-day cataract surgery and returning home would be classified as outpatient.

Diagnosis Reporting

- **Inpatient Coding**:
  - Allows coding of uncertain diagnoses documented at discharge as "probable," "suspected," or "likely."
  - *Example*: If a discharged patient's records state "probable myocardial infarction," it is coded as if confirmed.
- **Outpatient Coding**:
  - Requires coding only confirmed diagnoses; if uncertain, code the presenting symptoms.
  - *Example*: A patient presenting with chest pain but without a definitive diagnosis would have "chest pain" coded.

Documentation Focus

- **Inpatient Coding**:
  - Encompasses comprehensive documentation of the entire hospital stay, including all treatments and daily progress.
  - *Example*: A patient's record includes admission notes, surgical reports, daily physician updates, and discharge summary.
- **Outpatient Coding**:
  - Centers on specific encounters or visits, detailing the services provided during that time.
  - *Example*: Documentation for a patient receiving a flu shot would include the visit note and vaccine administration details.

Reimbursement Methodologies

- **Inpatient Coding**:
  - Uses the Inpatient Prospective Payment System (IPPS), with payments based on Diagnosis-Related Groups (DRGs).
  - *Example*: A patient undergoing hip replacement surgery is assigned a DRG that determines the hospital's reimbursement rate.
- **Outpatient Coding**:
  - Operates under the Outpatient Prospective Payment System (OPPS), utilizing Ambulatory Payment Classifications (APCs).
  - *Example*: A patient receiving outpatient chemotherapy is assigned an APC corresponding to the treatment provided.

Understanding these distinctions is crucial for accurate medical coding, ensuring compliance and appropriate reimbursement in healthcare settings.

Scenario Comparison: Identify Whether Each Example Belongs to Inpatient or Outpatient Coding

Instructions

Read each scenario carefully and determine if it falls under **inpatient** or **outpatient** coding.

Scenarios

1. A patient is admitted to the hospital for three days due to uncontrolled diabetes and receives IV insulin therapy.
    Answer: _____
2. A patient visits the emergency department for a sprained ankle, receives an X-ray and a brace, then is discharged the same day.
    Answer: _____
3. A patient undergoes an elective knee replacement surgery and stays in the hospital for two nights before discharge.
    Answer: _____
4. A patient visits a dermatologist for a routine skin check and removal of a suspicious mole in the same visit.
    Answer: _____
5. A patient is admitted for pneumonia treatment with IV antibiotics and continuous **monitoring for five days.**
    Answer: _____
6. A patient has a scheduled colonoscopy at an outpatient surgery center and is discharged after the procedure.
    Answer: _____
7. A pregnant woman is admitted for labor and delivery, staying in the hospital for two days before being discharged with her newborn.
    Answer: _____
8. A patient visits a cardiology clinic for a follow-up on hypertension management and medication adjustment.
    Answer: _____
9. A patient undergoes laparoscopic gallbladder removal and is sent home the same day.
    Answer: _____
10. A patient is admitted following a severe car accident, requiring multiple surgeries and intensive care for over a week.
    Answer: _____

Answer Key for Inpatient vs Outpatient Coding:

1. **Inpatient** – The patient was admitted for three days for diabetes management.
2. **Outpatient** – The patient was treated in the emergency department and discharged the same day.
3. **Inpatient** – The patient stayed in the hospital for two nights after knee replacement surgery.
4. **Outpatient** – The patient had a same-day dermatology visit and minor procedure.
5. **Inpatient** – The patient required hospitalization for pneumonia treatment over several days.
6. **Outpatient** – The colonoscopy was performed in an outpatient surgery center, and the patient was discharged the same day.
7. **Inpatient** – Labor and delivery require hospital admission and a multi-day stay.
8. **Outpatient** – The cardiology visit was a follow-up appointment without admission.
9. **Outpatient** – Laparoscopic gallbladder removal was performed as a same-day procedure.
10. **Inpatient** – The patient required prolonged hospitalization and multiple surgeries due to a severe car accident.

Common Medical Specialties

The medical field encompasses a wide range of specialties, each focusing on specific areas of patient care. Below is a list of common medical specialties:

- **Allergy and Immunology**: Focuses on diagnosing and treating allergic conditions and immune system disorders.
- **Anesthesiology**: Involves the administration of anesthesia and monitoring of patients during surgical procedures.
- **Cardiology**: Specializes in diagnosing and treating heart and blood vessel disorders.
- **Dermatology**: Deals with conditions related to the skin, hair, and nails.
- **Emergency Medicine**: Provides immediate care for acute illnesses and injuries.
- **Endocrinology**: Focuses on hormone-related disorders, including diabetes and thyroid diseases.
- **Gastroenterology**: Addresses diseases of the digestive system, including the stomach and intestines.
- **Hematology**: Concerns the study and treatment of blood disorders.
- **Infectious Disease**: Specializes in diagnosing and managing infections caused by bacteria, viruses, fungi, and parasites.
- **Internal Medicine**: Provides comprehensive care for adults, managing a wide range of medical conditions.
- **Nephrology**: Focuses on kidney function and related diseases.
- **Neurology**: Deals with disorders of the nervous system, including the brain and spinal cord.
- **Obstetrics and Gynecology (OB/GYN)**: Covers women's reproductive health, including pregnancy and childbirth.
- **Oncology**: Specializes in the diagnosis and treatment of cancer.
- **Ophthalmology**: Focuses on eye health, including vision care and eye surgeries.
- **Orthopedics**: Addresses conditions involving the musculoskeletal system, including bones and joints.
- **Otolaryngology (ENT)**: Deals with disorders of the ear, nose, and throat.
- **Pediatrics**: Provides medical care for infants, children, and adolescents.
- **Psychiatry**: Focuses on the diagnosis and treatment of mental health disorders.
- **Pulmonology**: Specializes in respiratory system disorders, including lung diseases.
- **Radiology**: Utilizes imaging techniques to diagnose and treat various conditions.
- **Rheumatology**: Deals with rheumatic diseases affecting joints and connective tissues.
- **Surgery**: Involves operative procedures to treat diseases, injuries, or deformities.
- **Urology**: Focuses on urinary tract disorders and male reproductive health.

Each specialty plays a vital role in delivering comprehensive healthcare, addressing specific patient needs through specialized knowledge and skills.

Cardiology: Case Examples with Relevant ICD-10 Codes

Case 1: Acute Myocardial Infarction (AMI)

- **Patient Details**: A 58-year-old male presents with severe chest pain radiating to the left arm, accompanied by shortness of breath and diaphoresis.
- **Examination Findings**: Electrocardiogram (ECG) shows ST-segment elevation in the anterior leads. Cardiac biomarkers are elevated.
- **Assessment**: ST-elevation myocardial infarction (STEMI) involving the left anterior descending coronary artery.
- ICD-10-CM **Code**: I21.02 – ST elevation (STEMI) myocardial infarction involving left anterior descending coronary artery.

Case 2: Chronic Heart Failure

- **Patient Details**: A 72-year-old female with a history of hypertension and diabetes mellitus reports progressive dyspnea on exertion and lower extremity edema.
- **Examination Findings**: Echocardiogram reveals a left ventricular ejection fraction (LVEF) of 35%, indicating systolic dysfunction.
- **Assessment**: Chronic systolic (congestive) heart failure.
- ICD-10-CM **Code**: I50.22 – Chronic systolic (congestive) heart failure.

Case 3: Atrial Fibrillation

- **Patient Details**: A 65-year-old male experiences palpitations, fatigue, and occasional dizziness.
- **Examination Findings**: ECG demonstrates an irregularly irregular rhythm without distinct P waves, consistent with atrial fibrillation.
- **Assessment**: Chronic atrial fibrillation.
- ICD-10-CM **Code**: I48.2 – Chronic atrial fibrillation.

Case 4: Hypertensive Heart Disease with Heart Failure

- **Patient Details**: A 60-year-old female with a long-standing history of uncontrolled hypertension presents with shortness of breath and fatigue.
- **Examination Findings**: Echocardiogram shows left ventricular hypertrophy and diastolic dysfunction.
- **Assessment**: Hypertensive heart disease with heart failure.
- ICD-10-CM **Code**: I11.0 – Hypertensive heart disease with heart failure.

Case 5: Unstable Angina

- **Patient Details**: A 70-year-old male reports chest pain at rest that has increased in frequency and severity over the past 48 hours.
- **Examination Findings**: ECG shows ST-segment depression in multiple leads; cardiac enzymes are within normal limits.
- **Assessment**: Unstable angina.
- ICD-10-CM **Code**: I20.0 – Unstable angina.

Case 6: Ventricular Tachycardia

- **Patient Details**: A 55-year-old male with a history of myocardial infarction experiences episodes of rapid heartbeats, dizziness, and near-syncope.
- **Examination Findings**: ECG during symptoms reveals wide-complex tachycardia at a rate of 160 beats per minute.
- **Assessment**: Sustained ventricular tachycardia.
- ICD-10-CM **Code**: I47.2 – Ventricular tachycardia.

Case 7: Mitral Valve Prolapse

- **Patient Details**: A 45-year-old female presents with palpitations and atypical chest pain.
- **Examination Findings**: Auscultation reveals a mid-systolic click followed by a late systolic murmur; echocardiogram confirms mitral valve prolapse.
- **Assessment**: Nonrheumatic mitral valve prolapse.
- ICD-10-CM **Code**: I34.1 – Nonrheumatic mitral (valve) prolapse.

Case 8: Peripheral Artery Disease

- **Patient Details**: A 68-year-old male complains of cramping pain in the calves after walking short distances, which is relieved by rest.
- **Examination Findings**: Diminished dorsalis pedis pulses bilaterally; ankle-brachial index (ABI) of 0.65.
- **Assessment**: Atherosclerosis of native arteries of the extremities with intermittent claudication.
- ICD-10-CM **Code**: I70.213 – Atherosclerosis of native arteries of extremities with intermittent claudication, bilateral legs.

Case 9: Acute Pericarditis

- **Patient Details**: A 50-year-old female presents with sharp, pleuritic chest pain that improves when sitting up and leaning forward.
- **Examination Findings**: Pericardial friction rub audible on auscultation; ECG shows diffuse ST-segment elevations.
- **Assessment**: Acute pericarditis.
- ICD-10-CM **Code**: I30.9 – Acute pericarditis, unspecified.

Case 10: Cardiomyopathy

- **Patient Details**: A 62-year-old male with a history of alcohol abuse presents with fatigue, dyspnea, and peripheral edema.
- **Examination Findings**: Echocardiogram reveals dilated ventricles with reduced systolic function.
- **Assessment**: Dilated cardiomyopathy.
- ICD-10-CM **Code**: I42.0 – Dilated cardiomyopathy.

These case examples illustrate common cardiovascular conditions and their corresponding ICD-10-CM codes, helping coders accurately document diagnoses and ensure compliance with coding guidelines. Mastering these cases enhances proficiency in cardiology coding and improves healthcare data accuracy.

Orthopedics: Focus on Fractures, Injuries, and Surgeries

Cancer Diagnosis Coding

- **Active Cancer Diagnosis**:
  - Use ICD-10-CM codes from the **C00-D49** range to specify the type and location of the malignancy.
  - Example: **C50.912** – Malignant neoplasm of unspecified site of left female breast.
- **Historical Cancer Diagnosis**:
  - When the cancer has been eradicated, and the patient is no longer receiving treatment, use codes from category **Z85** to indicate a personal history of malignant neoplasm.
  - Example: **Z85.3** – Personal history of malignant neoplasm of breast.
- **Uncertain Behavior Neoplasms**:
  - For neoplasms whose behavior cannot be determined as benign or malignant, use codes from category **D48**.
  - Example: **D48.5** – Neoplasm of uncertain behavior of skin.

Cancer Treatment Coding

- **Chemotherapy**:
  - Report encounters for chemotherapy using ICD-10-CM code **Z51.11** – Encounter for antineoplastic chemotherapy.
  - Administration of chemotherapy is coded with **CPT** codes ranging from **96401** to **96549**, depending on the specific service provided.
- **Radiation Therapy**:
  - Use ICD-10-CM code **Z51.0** – Encounter for antineoplastic radiation therapy, for patients receiving radiation treatment.
  - Radiation therapy services are reported with **CPT** codes **77261** to **77799**, covering various aspects of treatment planning and delivery.
- **Immunotherapy**:
  - Encounters for immunotherapy are coded with ICD-10-CM code **Z51.12** – Encounter for antineoplastic immunotherapy.
  - Administration services are reported using **CPT** codes such as **96365** for intravenous infusion.
- **Surgical Treatment**:
  - Assign ICD-10-CM codes corresponding to the specific malignancy being addressed surgically.
  - Surgical procedures are reported with **CPT** codes ranging from **10004** to **69990**, depending on the procedure performed.

Key Considerations

- **Sequencing**:
  - When a patient is admitted for the purpose of receiving chemotherapy, immunotherapy, or radiation therapy, the appropriate **Z51** code should be listed as the principal diagnosis.
  - The malignancy for which the therapy is being administered should be coded as a secondary diagnosis.
- **Metastatic Sites**:
  - Code each metastatic site separately using ICD-10-CM codes from categories **C77** to **C79**, indicating secondary malignant neoplasms.
  - Example: **C78.7** – Secondary malignant neoplasm of liver and intrahepatic bile duct.
- **Complications**:
  - If a patient develops complications related to cancer treatment, such as anemia due to chemotherapy, assign codes for the specific complication in addition to the treatment code.
  - Example: **D64.81** – Anemia due to antineoplastic chemotherapy.

Accurate coding in oncology requires detailed documentation of the cancer's type, location, behavior, and the treatments administered. Staying current with coding guidelines ensures proper billing and optimal patient care.

Interactive Worksheet: Solve Specialty-Specific Coding Problems for Each Category

Instructions

Read each case scenario and assign the correct ICD-10-CM code(s). Consider primary and secondary diagnoses, treatment plans, and complications when coding.

Cardiology Case

Scenario: A 65-year-old male presents with chest pain and shortness of breath. An ECG confirms an ST-elevation myocardial infarction (STEMI) in the anterior wall. The patient undergoes coronary angioplasty.

Question:

- Assign the correct ICD-10-CM code for the myocardial infarction.
- Assign the appropriate procedure code for coronary angioplasty.

Answer: _____

Orthopedics Case

Scenario: A 45-year-old female falls down the stairs and sustains a closed displaced fracture of the right distal radius. The fracture is treated with closed reduction and casting.

Question:

- Assign the correct ICD-10-CM code for the fracture.

- Assign the procedure code for the closed reduction treatment.

Answer: _____

Oncology Case

Scenario: A 58-year-old female with stage II breast cancer of the right breast undergoes chemotherapy. She has no history of previous cancer treatment.

Question:

- Assign the correct ICD-10-CM code for the breast cancer.
- Assign the ICD-10-CM code for the chemotherapy encounter.

Answer: _____

Neurology Case

Scenario: A 72-year-old male with a history of hypertension and diabetes is admitted with left-sided weakness and slurred speech. CT scan confirms an acute ischemic stroke affecting the right middle cerebral artery.

Question:

- Assign the ICD-10-CM code for the stroke.
- Assign any secondary codes related to the patient's conditions.

Answer: _____

Endocrinology Case

Scenario: A 50-year-old female with a long history of uncontrolled type 2 diabetes mellitus presents with diabetic nephropathy. Lab results confirm elevated creatinine levels and proteinuria.

Question:

- Assign the ICD-10-CM code for the diabetes diagnosis.
- Assign the ICD-10-CM code for the associated nephropathy.

Answer: _____

Pulmonology Case

Scenario: A 65-year-old male with a 50-year smoking history presents with chronic obstructive pulmonary disease (COPD) exacerbation. He requires oxygen therapy and nebulized bronchodilators in the emergency department.

Question:

- Assign the ICD-10-CM code for COPD with exacerbation.
- Assign the ICD-10-CM code for the patient's smoking history.

Answer: _____

Gastroenterology Case

Scenario: A 40-year-old female is diagnosed with a bleeding gastric ulcer. An upper endoscopy (EGD) confirms an active ulcer with hemorrhage.

Question:

- Assign the ICD-10-CM code for the gastric ulcer with bleeding.
- Assign the procedure code for the endoscopy.

Answer: _____

Obstetrics & Gynecology Case

Scenario: A 32-year-old pregnant female at 28 weeks gestation is diagnosed with gestational hypertension without proteinuria.

Question:

- Assign the ICD-10-CM code for the gestational hypertension.
- Assign the ICD-10-CM code for the pregnancy status.

Answer: _____

Psychiatry Case

Scenario: A 22-year-old male with generalized anxiety disorder (GAD) is seen for worsening symptoms, including insomnia and panic attacks.

Question:

- Assign the ICD-10-CM code for generalized anxiety disorder.
- Assign an additional code for the patient's sleep disturbances.

Answer: _____

Answer Key for Interactive Worksheet

Cardiology Case

- **I21.09** – ST elevation (STEMI) myocardial infarction involving other coronary artery of anterior wall
- **02703ZZ** – Percutaneous transluminal coronary angioplasty (PTCA)

Orthopedics Case

- **S52.501A** – Unspecified fracture of the lower end of the right radius, initial encounter for closed fracture
- **24505** – Closed reduction of distal radius fracture with manipulation

Oncology Case

- **C50.911** – Malignant neoplasm of unspecified site of right female breast
- **Z51.11** – Encounter for antineoplastic chemotherapy

Neurology Case

- **I63.511** – Cerebral infarction due to occlusion or stenosis of right middle cerebral artery
- **E11.9** – Type 2 diabetes mellitus without complications
- **I10** – Essential (primary) hypertension

Endocrinology Case

- **E11.22** – Type 2 diabetes mellitus with diabetic chronic kidney disease
- **N18.9** – Chronic kidney disease, unspecified

Pulmonology Case

- **J44.1** – Chronic obstructive pulmonary disease with (acute) exacerbation
- **Z87.891** – Personal history of nicotine dependence

Gastroenterology Case

- **K25.4** – Gastric ulcer with hemorrhage
- **43235** – Esophagogastroduodenoscopy (EGD) with biopsy

Obstetrics & Gynecology Case

- **O13.3** – Gestational hypertension without significant proteinuria, third trimester
- **Z3A.28** – 28 weeks gestation of pregnancy

Psychiatry Case

F41.1 – Generalized anxiety disorder (GAD)
- **G47.00** – Insomnia, unspecified

Pediatric and Geriatric Coding

Geriatric Coding

- **Age-Specific Codes**:
  - Certain ICD-10-CM codes are designated specifically for patients aged 0–17 years. These codes address conditions unique to or primarily occurring in children. For example, **E30.8** denotes "Other disorders of puberty," applicable to pediatric patients.
- **Common Pediatric Diagnoses**:
  - **Acute Pharyngitis**: Inflammation of the pharynx, often leading to sore throat.
  - **Otitis Media**: Middle ear infection prevalent among young children.
  - **Asthma**: Chronic respiratory condition characterized by airway inflammation and bronchoconstriction.
  - **Gastroenteritis**: Inflammation of the stomach and intestines, leading to vomiting and diarrhea.
- **Documentation Tips**:
  - **Specificity**: Include detailed information such as anatomical location, severity, and associated complications.
  - **Growth and Development**: Document any deviations from typical developmental milestones, as these are crucial for accurate coding and treatment planning.
  - **Vaccination Status**: Record immunization history, especially when diagnosing vaccine-preventable diseases.

Geriatric Coding

- **Age-Specific Codes**:
  - Certain conditions have codes applicable to older adults. For instance, **R54** represents "Age-related physical debility," encompassing terms like frailty and senile asthenia.
- **Common Geriatric Diagnoses**:
  - **Dementia**: Chronic cognitive decline affecting memory and daily functioning.
  - **Osteoporosis**: Bone density loss increasing fracture risk.
  - **Arthritis**: Joint inflammation causing pain and stiffness.
  - **Hypertension**: Elevated blood pressure requiring regular monitoring.
- **Documentation Tips**:
  - **Comorbidities**: Thoroughly document all existing conditions, as multiple comorbidities are common and impact management plans.
  - **Functional Status**: Assess and record the patient's ability to perform activities of daily living, which influences care decisions.
  - **Medication Review**: Regularly document all medications, considering polypharmacy risks prevalent in geriatric patients.
- **Recent Updates**:
  - As of January 1, 2025, new **ICD-10-PCS** codes have been introduced, effective for discharges and patient encounters from April 1, 2025, to September 30, 2025. These updates include 50 new procedure codes pertinent to various specialties, including geriatrics.

Accurate coding in both pediatric and geriatric populations necessitates attention to age-specific conditions, detailed documentation, and staying informed about the latest coding updates to ensure optimal patient care and compliance.

Top 10 Mistakes in ICD-10-CM Coding

Accurate ICD-10-CM coding is essential for proper documentation and reimbursement in healthcare. However, common mistakes can lead to claim denials and compliance issues. Here are the top 10 errors to avoid:

1. **Using Outdated Codes**:
   - Regularly update your ICD-10-CM code sets and guidelines to reflect the latest coding requirements. Using outdated codes leads to automatic denials.
2. **Lack of Specificity**:
   - ICD-10-CM codes often require specific details in the fourth and fifth digits. Using truncated codes (missing these details) is a common error that guarantees claim denial.
3. **Incorrect Sequencing of Codes**:
   - Not following instructions for sequencing codes is incorrect coding and non-compliant with HIPAA. Ensure that primary and secondary diagnoses are ordered correctly.
4. **Confusing Similar Characters**:
   - Mixing up similar-looking numbers and letters, such as '0' (zero) and 'O' or '1' (one) and 'I', can lead to incorrect coding. Pay close attention to these characters to prevent errors.
5. **Omitting Laterality and Specificity**:
   - ICD-10-CM emphasizes the need for detailed documentation, including the side of the body affected (laterality) and specific disease processes. Ensure that such details are included to select the most accurate code.
6. **Neglecting Code Updates and Guidelines**:
   - ICD-10-CM codes and guidelines are updated annually. Failing to stay current with these changes can result in the use of obsolete codes and non-compliance. Regularly review official updates to maintain accuracy.
7. **Improper Use of Combination Codes**:
   - ICD-10-CM includes combination codes that capture multiple components of a diagnosis. Using multiple codes when a combination code exists, or vice versa, can lead to redundancy or incomplete coding.
8. **Inadequate Documentation for Code Selection**:
   - Accurate coding relies on thorough and precise documentation. Insufficient detail can lead to the selection of unspecified codes, which may not reflect the patient's condition accurately. Encourage comprehensive documentation practices.
9. **Misapplication of Excludes Notes**:
   - ICD-10-CM uses 'Excludes1' and 'Excludes2' notes to indicate when conditions cannot be coded together or when they may be reported together under certain circumstances. Misinterpreting these notes can lead to coding errors.
10. **Overlooking External Cause Codes**:
    - For injuries and certain conditions, external cause codes provide context about how the injury or condition occurred. Omitting these codes when required can result in incomplete documentation.

By being aware of these common mistakes and implementing thorough documentation and regular training, healthcare providers can enhance coding accuracy, reduce claim denials, and ensure compliance with current ICD-10-CM guidelines.

Mini Quiz: Differentiate Between Pediatric and Geriatric Coding Rules

Instructions

Read each statement carefully and determine whether it applies to pediatric coding, geriatric coding, or both.

Questions

1. This category of patients may have vaccine-preventable diseases documented in their medical history.
   Answer: _____
2. Coding must account for multiple chronic conditions and comorbidities that impact treatment decisions.
   Answer: _____
3. Growth and developmental milestones are an essential part of documentation.
   Answer: _____
4. ICD-10-CM code R54 is commonly used to describe conditions in this patient group.
   Answer: _____
5. Conditions like failure to thrive (FTT) are more commonly coded in this population.
   Answer: _____
6. Z00.129 is used for a routine health examination in this group without abnormal findings.
   Answer: _____
7. Polypharmacy (the use of multiple medications) is a common concern in coding for this population.
   Answer: _____
8. Osteoporosis and fall-related injuries frequently appear in medical records.
   Answer: _____
9. ICD-10-CM codes for congenital disorders are most frequently assigned in this category.
   Answer: _____
10. Coding guidelines emphasize tracking immunization status and preventive screenings.
    Answer: _____

Answer Key for Pediatric and Geriatric Coding Rules

1. **Pediatric** – Vaccine-preventable diseases are a key consideration in pediatric coding.
2. **Geriatric** – Multiple chronic conditions and comorbidities are more common in older adults.
3. **Pediatric** – Growth and developmental milestones are essential for tracking a child's health.
4. **Geriatric** – ICD-10-CM code **R54** refers to age-related physical debility.
5. **Pediatric** – Failure to thrive (FTT) is primarily diagnosed in infants and young children.
6. **Pediatric** – **Z00.129** is used for routine child health exams without abnormalities.
7. **Geriatric** – Polypharmacy is a significant issue in older adults due to multiple prescriptions.
8. **Geriatric** – Osteoporosis and fall-related injuries frequently occur in elderly patients.
9. **Pediatric** – Congenital disorders are primarily coded for newborns and young children.
10. **Both** – Immunization status is crucial in pediatric care, while preventive screenings are important in both age groups.

Error Analysis Exercise: Identify and Correct Errors in Provided Examples

Instructions

Review each coding scenario below and identify any **errors** in the assigned ICD-10-CM codes. Determine the correct coding approach based on documentation, sequencing, and specificity.

Case 1: Incorrect Code Selection

Scenario: A 45-year-old female presents with acute exacerbation of chronic obstructive pulmonary disease (COPD) due to influenza. The coder assigned:

- **J44.1** – COPD with (acute) exacerbation
- **J11.1** – Influenza with other respiratory manifestations

Question:

- Identify the error in the coding.
- What should the correct ICD-10-CM code(s) be?

Case 2: Incorrect Sequencing

Scenario: A 60-year-old male with a history of hypertension and chronic kidney disease (CKD) stage **3** presents for routine follow-up. The coder assigned:

- **N18.3** – Chronic kidney disease, stage 3
- **I10** – Essential (primary) hypertension

Question:

- Identify the sequencing issue.
- What is the correct order for these codes?

Case 3: Missing Laterality

Scenario: A 35-year-old female suffers a traumatic fracture of the right distal tibia after falling down the stairs. The coder assigned:

- **S82.209A** – Unspecified fracture of the tibia, initial encounter

Question:

- What specific detail is missing in this code assignment?
- How should the correct code be selected?

Case 4: Overuse of Unspecified Codes

Scenario: A 50-year-old male is diagnosed with type 2 diabetes mellitus with diabetic neuropathy, but the coder assigned:

- **E11.9** – Type 2 diabetes mellitus without complications

Question:

- What error did the coder make?
- What should be the correct code to capture the full diagnosis?

Case 5: Excludes1 Note Violation

Scenario: A 28-year-old female is diagnosed with acute pyelonephritis and a lower urinary tract infection (UTI). The coder assigned:

- **N10** – Acute pyelonephritis
- **N39.0** – Urinary tract infection, site not specified

Question:

- Why is this code combination incorrect?
- What correction should be made based on Excludes1 rules?

Case 6: Omission of External Cause Code

Scenario: A 40-year-old male is seen in the emergency department for a left wrist sprain due to a fall from a ladder at work. The coder assigned:

- **S63.502A** – Sprain of unspecified ligament of left wrist, initial encounter

Question:

- What important detail is missing in this coding?
- What additional code(s) should be included for proper reporting?

Case 7: Incorrect Code for Pregnancy Condition

Scenario: A 32-year-old pregnant female at 28 weeks gestation is diagnosed with gestational hypertension. The coder assigned:

- **I10** – Essential (primary) hypertension

Question:

- Why is this code incorrect for this diagnosis?
- What should be the correct code reflecting the pregnancy condition?

Case 8: Using an Outdated Code

Scenario: A 70-year-old male presents with senile osteoporosis with a recent pathological fracture of the vertebra. The coder assigned:

- **M81.0** – Age-related osteoporosis without current pathological fracture

Question:

- What is incorrect about this code selection?
- What should be coded instead to accurately capture the fracture?

Case 9: Failure to Assign Combination Code

Scenario: A 55-year-old female with hypertensive heart disease and heart failure was coded as:

- **I10** – Essential (primary) hypertension
- **I50.22** – Chronic systolic (congestive) heart failure

Question:

- What combination code should have been used instead?
- Why is the current coding approach incorrect?

Case 10: Unnecessary Use of Separate Codes

Scenario: A 45-year-old male is diagnosed with chronic gout with tophi in his left ankle. The coder assigned:

- **M10.072** – Gout, left ankle
- **M14.672** – Tophus, left ankle

Question:

- Why is this coding approach incorrect?
- What is the correct way to assign a code for chronic tophaceous gout?

Answer Key for Error Analysis Exercise:

Case 1: Incorrect Code Selection

- **Error: J11.1** (Influenza with other respiratory manifestations) is incorrect because the flu has been confirmed.
- **Correct Code: J44.0** (COPD with acute lower respiratory infection) and **J09.X2** (Influenza due to identified novel influenza A virus with other respiratory manifestations).

Case 2: Incorrect Sequencing

- **Error: I10** (Hypertension) is listed after **N18.3** (CKD Stage 3), but hypertensive CKD requires a combination code.
- **Correct Code Order:**
  - **I12.9** – Hypertensive chronic kidney disease with stage 1-4 CKD
  - **N18.3** – Chronic kidney disease, stage 3

Case 3: Missing Laterality

- **Error: S82.209A** (Unspecified fracture of the tibia) does not specify right or left side.
- **Correct Code: S82.201A** (Unspecified fracture of shaft of right tibia, initial encounter).

Case 4: Overuse of Unspecified Codes

- **Error: E11.9** (Type 2 diabetes mellitus without complications) does not reflect the neuropathy.
- **Correct Code: E11.40** (Type 2 diabetes mellitus with diabetic neuropathy, unspecified).

Case 5: Excludes1 Note Violation

- **Error: N10** (Acute pyelonephritis) and **N39.0** (UTI) cannot be coded together because acute pyelonephritis includes lower urinary tract infections.
- **Correct Code: N10** (Acute pyelonephritis) alone is sufficient.

Case 6: Omission of External Cause Code

- **Error:** Missing external cause codes for the injury mechanism and place of occurrence.
- **Correct Codes:**
  - **S63.502A** – Sprain of unspecified ligament of left wrist, initial encounter
  - **W11.XXXA** – Fall from ladder, initial encounter
  - **Y92.62** – Place of occurrence: Worksite

Case 7: Incorrect Code for Pregnancy Condition

- **Error: I10** (Primary hypertension) does not apply to pregnancy-related hypertension.
- **Correct Code: O13.3** (Gestational hypertension without significant proteinuria, third trimester).

Case 8: Using an Outdated Code

- **Error: M81.0** (Age-related osteoporosis without fracture) does not reflect the current fracture.
- **Correct Code: M80.08XA** (Age-related osteoporosis with current pathological fracture, vertebra, initial encounter).

Case 9: Failure to Assign Combination Code

- **Error:** Separate codes for hypertension and heart failure were used instead of a combination code.
- **Correct Code: I11.0** (Hypertensive heart disease with heart failure).

Case 10: Unnecessary Use of Separate Codes

- **Error: M10.072** (Gout) and **M14.672** (Tophus) should not be coded separately when a **combination code** exists.
- **Correct Code: M1A.0720** (Chronic gout with tophi, left ankle, without chronic kidney disease).

Troubleshooting Guide for ICD-10-CM Coding

Accurate ICD-10-CM coding is essential for proper documentation and reimbursement in healthcare. To assist coders in navigating common challenges, here is a troubleshooting guide:

- **Regularly Update Code Sets**:
  - Ensure that your ICD-10-CM code sets and guidelines are current. Using outdated codes can lead to claim denials. The Centers for Medicare & Medicaid Services (CMS) periodically release updates; for instance, 50 new ICD-10-PCS codes were announced, effective April 1, 2025.
- **Ensure Specificity in Coding**:
  - Assign codes to the highest level of specificity based on the medical record. Avoid using unspecified codes when detailed information is available. For example, laterality (left, right, bilateral) should be specified when applicable.
- **Verify Code Selection**:
  - Always cross-reference codes from the Alphabetic Index with the Tabular List to confirm accuracy. This practice helps ensure that all required characters and extensions are included.
- **Understand Excludes Notes**:
  - Familiarize yourself with 'Excludes1' and 'Excludes2' notes in the Tabular List. 'Excludes1' indicates that the excluded code should not be used simultaneously, while 'Excludes2' allows for concurrent coding if documentation supports both conditions.
- **Avoid Assumptions Without Documentation**:
  - Do not code conditions labeled as 'probable,' 'suspected,' or 'rule out.' Only code diagnoses confirmed by the provider. If a definitive diagnosis is not established, code the presenting signs or symptoms.
- **Utilize Combination Codes Appropriately**:
  - When a single code describes multiple aspects of a condition, use combination codes to capture the full clinical picture without redundancy.
- **Stay Informed on Coding Guidelines**:
  - Regularly review the ICD-10-CM Official Guidelines for Coding and Reporting to stay updated on conventions and instructions. These guidelines are essential for accurate code assignment.
- **Ensure Accurate Code Sequencing**:
  - Follow the ICD-10-CM guidelines for sequencing codes, especially when dealing with multiple diagnoses. Proper sequencing affects reimbursement and reflects the patient's clinical status accurately.
- **Conduct Regular Audits and Training**:
  - Implement routine audits to identify and correct coding errors. Continuous education and training help coders stay proficient and up-to-date with coding standards.

By adhering to these practices, healthcare providers can enhance coding accuracy, reduce claim denials, and ensure compliance with current ICD-10-CM guidelines.

Q&A Worksheet: Practice Troubleshooting Common Challenges

Instructions

Review each scenario and answer the corresponding question. Identify coding errors, documentation issues, or sequencing problems and provide the correct approach.

Case 1: Incorrect Code Selection

Scenario: A 60-year-old female presents with acute exacerbation of chronic obstructive pulmonary disease (COPD) due to pneumonia. The coder assigned:

- **J44.1** – COPD with (acute) exacerbation
- **J18.9** – Pneumonia, unspecified organism

Question:

- Identify the coding mistake in this scenario.
- What should be the correct ICD-10-CM code(s)?

Case 2: Incorrect Code Sequencing

Scenario: A 70-year-old male with diabetes mellitus and peripheral neuropathy presents for routine management. The coder assigned:

- **E11.9** – Type 2 diabetes mellitus without complications
- **G62.9** – Polyneuropathy, unspecified

Question:

- What sequencing error exists in this case?
- What is the correct way to code diabetic neuropathy?

Case 3: Unspecified Diagnosis Used

Scenario: A 45-year-old female is diagnosed with osteoarthritis of the right knee, but the coder assigned:

- **M19.90** – Osteoarthritis, unspecified site, unspecified type

Question:

- What specific detail is missing?
- How should the correct code be selected?

Case 4: Omission of External Cause Code

Scenario: A 35-year-old male was injured in a motor vehicle accident, sustaining a concussion without loss of consciousness. The coder assigned:

- **S06.0X0A** – Concussion without loss of consciousness, initial encounter

Question:

- What important detail is missing from the documentation?
- What additional code(s) should be included?

Case 5: Pregnancy-Related Diagnosis Coded Incorrectly

Scenario: A 28-year-old pregnant female at 32 weeks gestation is diagnosed with gestational diabetes controlled with diet. The coder assigned:

- **E11.9** – Type 2 diabetes mellitus without complications

Question:

- Why is this code incorrect for a pregnancy-related diabetes diagnosis?
- What should be the correct ICD-10-CM code?

Case 6: Using an Outdated Code

Scenario: A 75-year-old male presents with age-related osteoporosis with a recent pathological vertebral fracture. The coder assigned:

- **M81.0** – Age-related osteoporosis without current pathological fracture

Question:

- What is incorrect about this code selection?
- What should be coded instead?

Case 7: Missing Laterality Information

Scenario: A 50-year-old female has been diagnosed with carpal tunnel syndrome but the coder assigned:

- **G56.00** – Carpal tunnel syndrome, unspecified upper limb

Question:

- What information is missing in this coding?
- How should the correct code be selected?

Case 8: Failure to Use a Combination Code

Scenario: A 55-year-old male with hypertensive heart disease and heart failure was coded as:

- **I10** – Essential hypertension
- **I50.9** – Heart failure, unspecified

Question:

- What coding error was made in this scenario?
- What should be the correct ICD-10-CM code?

Case 9: Excludes1 Note Violation

Scenario: A 40-year-old female is diagnosed with acute sinusitis and chronic sinusitis. The coder assigned:

- **J01.90** – Acute sinusitis, unspecified
- **J32.9** – Chronic sinusitis, unspecified

Question:

- Why is this code combination incorrect?
- What should be coded instead based on Excludes1 rules?

Case 10: Overuse of Unspecified Codes

Scenario: A 30-year-old male is diagnosed with benign prostatic hyperplasia with lower urinary tract symptoms (LUTS). The coder assigned:

- **N40.0** – Benign prostatic hyperplasia without lower urinary tract symptoms

Question:

- What error did the coder make in this scenario?
- What is the correct way to document this condition?

Answer Key for Troubleshooting Guide

Case 1: Incorrect Code Selection

- **Error: J44.1** (COPD with exacerbation) and **J18.9** (unspecified pneumonia) do not accurately capture the interaction between the two conditions.
- **Correct Codes:**
    - **J44.0** – COPD with lower respiratory infection.
    - **J18.9** – Pneumonia, unspecified organism.

Case 2: Incorrect Code Sequencing

- **Error:** The coder listed **E11.9** (diabetes without complications) instead of using a code that reflects the neuropathy.
- **Correct Code: E11.40** – Type 2 diabetes mellitus with diabetic neuropathy.

Case 3: Unspecified Diagnosis Used

- **Error: M19.90** (unspecified osteoarthritis) does not indicate the specific joint affected.
- **Correct Code: M17.11** – Unilateral primary osteoarthritis, right knee.

Case 4: Omission of External Cause Code

- **Error:** The coder did not include an external cause code to indicate how the injury occurred.
- **Correct Codes:**
    - **S06.0X0A** – Concussion without loss of consciousness, initial encounter.
    - **V43.52XA** – Driver injured in collision with another vehicle, initial encounter

Case 5: Pregnancy-Related Diagnosis Coded Incorrectly

- **Error: E11.9** is used for type 2 diabetes but does not apply to gestational diabetes.
- **Correct Code: O24.419** – Gestational diabetes mellitus in pregnancy, diet-controlled.

Case 6: Using an Outdated Code

- **Error: M81.0** (osteoporosis without current fracture) is incorrect because the patient has a **recent fracture**.
- **Correct Code: M80.08XA** – Age-related osteoporosis with current pathological fracture, vertebra, initial encounter.

Case 7: Missing Laterality Information

- **Error: G56.00** (unspecified carpal tunnel syndrome) does not indicate whether the right or left hand is affected.
- **Correct Code:**
  - **G56.01** – Carpal tunnel syndrome, right upper limb.
  - **G56.02** – Carpal tunnel syndrome, left upper limb (if applicable).

Case 8: Failure to Use a Combination Code

- **Error:** The coder used separate codes for hypertension and heart failure instead of a combination code.
- **Correct Code: I11.0** – Hypertensive heart disease with heart failure

Case 9: Excludes1 Note Violation

- **Error: J01.90** (acute sinusitis) and **J32.9** (chronic sinusitis) cannot be coded together due to Excludes1 rules.
- **Correct Code: J32.0** – Chronic maxillary sinusitis (or the specific type documented).

Case 10: Overuse of Unspecified Codes

- **Error: N40.0** (benign prostatic hyperplasia without symptoms) does not reflect the patient's **lower urinary tract symptoms (LUTS)**.
- **Correct Code: N40.1** – Benign prostatic hyperplasia with lower urinary tract symptoms.

QUESTION & ANSWERS

'What does ICD-10-CM **stand for?'**
'ICD-10-CM stands for International Classification of Diseases, 10th Revision, Clinical Modification. It is the standardized coding system used in the United States for diagnosing diseases and health conditions in outpatient and inpatient settings. It provides detailed codes that allow for greater specificity in medical documentation and billing.'

'How many characters can an ICD-10-CM **code have?'**
'An ICD-10-CM code can have between three and seven characters. The first character is always a letter, the second and third characters are numbers, and the fourth through seventh characters can be a mix of numbers and letters. The additional characters allow for more precise descriptions of the diagnosis, including laterality, severity, and any associated complications.'

'What does the letter "X" represent in an ICD-10-CM **code?'**
'The letter "X" is used as a placeholder in ICD-10-CM codes. It ensures the proper format and structure of the code when a future expansion may require additional specificity. It is commonly used in codes that require a seventh character but do not have a sixth-character requirement.'

'Which section of the ICD-10-CM **guidelines should be referenced first for general coding rules?'**
'The ICD-10-CM Official Guidelines for Coding and Reporting should always be referenced first. These guidelines, updated annually by the National Center for Health Statistics (NCHS) and the Centers for Medicare & Medicaid Services (CMS), provide essential rules on code selection, sequencing, and application in various healthcare settings.'

'What is an "Excludes1" note in ICD-10-CM?'
'An Excludes1 note means that two conditions cannot be coded together because they describe the same condition or a different condition that cannot coexist with the first. For example, if a code for congenital heart disease has an Excludes1 note for acquired heart disease, only one of those codes can be assigned to a patient's record, depending on the diagnosis.'

'If a physician documents "suspected pneumonia," can it be coded as pneumonia?'
'No, in outpatient settings, suspected, probable, or ruled-out diagnoses cannot be coded as confirmed conditions. Instead, the coder should report the signs and symptoms present at the time of the visit, such as cough, fever, or shortness of breath. However, in inpatient settings, suspected conditions documented at discharge may be coded as if they were confirmed.'

'What does laterality mean in ICD-10-CM?'
'Laterality refers to whether a condition affects the right, left, or both sides of the body. Many ICD-10-CM codes include laterality, requiring coders to specify whether a diagnosis applies to the left, right, or bilateral site. If the documentation does not specify laterality, an unspecified code should be used, though it may not be reimbursable in some cases.'

'What should be coded if a provider documents "abdominal pain, possible appendicitis" in an outpatient setting?'
'In an outpatient setting, only confirmed diagnoses should be coded. Since appendicitis is only suspected and not confirmed, the coder should report the symptom of abdominal pain using the appropriate ICD-10-CM code, such as R10.9 (unspecified abdominal pain).'

'Which section of ICD-10-CM **is used for social determinants of health (SDOH)?'**
'The Z codes (Z55-Z65) are used to report social determinants of health, such as housing instability, financial difficulties, education barriers, or food insecurity. These codes help document external factors that influence a patient's health status and access to care.'

'Can the same diagnosis code be reported multiple times for a single encounter?'
'No, the same ICD-10-CM diagnosis code should not be reported multiple times for a single encounter. If a patient has multiple sites affected by the same condition, the coder should check whether there is a code that includes multiple sites. If no such code exists, separate codes may be assigned for each affected site.'

'What is a combination code in ICD-10-CM?'
'A combination code is a single ICD-10-CM code that captures two or more conditions that commonly occur together or one condition with an associated complication. For example, E11.22 (Type 2 diabetes mellitus with chronic kidney disease) is a combination code that describes both diabetes and its related kidney disease.'

'What is the significance of a seventh character in ICD-10-CM?'
'The seventh character in ICD-10-CM is used in certain code categories, mainly in injury, fracture, and pregnancy-related codes, to provide more detail about the episode of care. The three most common seventh characters are "A" for the initial encounter, "D" for the subsequent encounter, and "S" for sequela (a complication or residual effect of an earlier condition).'

'What is the difference between Excludes1 and Excludes2 notes?'
'Excludes1 notes indicate that two conditions should never be coded together because they describe the same condition. Excludes2 notes mean that while the two conditions are not part of the same diagnosis, they may coexist and be reported together if the documentation supports it.'

'What is the correct way to code a diagnosis that is documented as "ruled out"?'
'If a diagnosis is documented as "ruled out," it should not be coded in the outpatient setting. Instead, the coder should report the symptoms or signs that led to the evaluation. In inpatient settings, ruled-out conditions should not be coded unless there is supporting documentation indicating a clinical reason for their inclusion.'

'How should a coder handle a medical record that lacks sufficient documentation for an accurate diagnosis code?'
'If a medical record lacks sufficient documentation, the coder should query the provider for clarification before selecting a code. Using an unspecified code may be necessary if the documentation remains incomplete, but it should only be done as a last resort.'

'What is the purpose of external cause codes?'
'External cause codes describe how an injury or condition occurred, such as a fall, motor vehicle accident, or exposure to a harmful substance. These codes are not primary diagnoses but provide additional context about an injury.'

'Are external cause codes required for all injuries?'
'While external cause codes are not mandatory for all injuries, they are highly recommended in cases involving trauma, accidents, or violence. Some payers may require them for reimbursement.'

'What does the seventh character "S" indicate in injury coding?'
'The seventh character "S" in injury coding signifies a sequela, meaning the patient is being treated for a complication or residual effect of an earlier injury. For example, a patient with chronic pain from a healed fracture would have a code ending in "S" to indicate the long-term effects of the original injury.'

'Which category is used to report pregnancy-related conditions?
'Pregnancy-related conditions are reported using codes from Chapter 15 (O00-O9A) of ICD-10-CM. These codes take priority over other codes unless the reason for the visit is unrelated to pregnancy.

'What is the correct way to code a newborn with meconium aspiration syndrome?
'The appropriate code is P24.01 (Meconium aspiration syndrome with respiratory symptoms), which falls under the perinatal conditions category.

'How should a coder report hypertension with chronic kidney disease?'
'Hypertension with chronic kidney disease should be reported using a combination code from category I12 (Hypertensive chronic kidney disease). The specific stage of chronic kidney disease should also be included using an additional code from category N18. For example, I12.9 (Hypertensive chronic kidney disease with stage 1-4 CKD) and N18.4 (Chronic kidney disease, stage 4) would be used together.'

'When coding diabetes with complications, should separate codes be assigned?'
'No, ICD-10-CM provides combination codes that describe both diabetes and its complications. For example, E11.22 (Type 2 diabetes mellitus with chronic kidney disease) captures both conditions in one code, eliminating the need for separate diagnosis codes.'

'What code should be assigned for a patient with stage 5 chronic kidney disease who is also on dialysis?'
'The correct code for stage 5 chronic kidney disease is N18.5. However, if the patient is on long-term dialysis, an additional code, Z99.2 (Dependence on renal dialysis), should be assigned to indicate ongoing treatment.'

'How should a coder report a patient with a history of breast cancer that has been treated and is no longer active?'
'If a patient has a history of breast cancer and is no longer receiving treatment, a history code should be used instead of an active cancer diagnosis. The correct code would be Z85.3 (Personal history of malignant neoplasm of breast).'

'When coding metastatic cancer, which site should be coded first?'
'The primary site of cancer should be coded first unless the reason for the visit is specifically to treat the metastatic site. If a patient has lung cancer that has spread to the liver, the primary code would be C34.90 (Malignant neoplasm of unspecified part of unspecified bronchus or lung), followed by C78.7 (Secondary malignant neoplasm of liver and intrahepatic bile duct).'

'How should a patient receiving chemotherapy be coded?'
'When a patient is undergoing chemotherapy, the primary diagnosis should be the appropriate Z code for the treatment encounter. The correct code would be Z51.11 (Encounter for antineoplastic chemotherapy). The malignancy being treated should also be coded as a secondary diagnosis.'

'What is the correct way to code failure to thrive in a child?'
'Failure to thrive in a pediatric patient should be reported using the code R62.51 (Failure to thrive, child). However, if the provider specifies neonatal failure to thrive, P92.6 (Failure to thrive in newborn) should be used instead.'

'What ICD-10-CM code is used to report age-related physical debility in an elderly patient?'
'The appropriate code for age-related physical debility or frailty in elderly patients is R54 (Age-related physical debility). This code should only be assigned when the physician explicitly documents frailty or general age-related weakness.'

'How should a coder report a patient who was injured in a fall from a ladder at work?'
'In addition to the primary injury diagnosis code, an external cause code should be assigned to specify how the injury occurred. The correct external cause code would be W11.XXXA (Fall from ladder, initial encounter), along with a place of occurrence code such as Y92.62 (Worksite, not specified).'

'What additional codes should be assigned when a patient is bitten by a dog?'
'The primary code should describe the injury itself, such as S51.851A (Open bite of right forearm, initial encounter). Additionally, an external cause code, W54.0XXA (Bitten by dog, initial encounter), should be assigned to document the cause of the injury.'

'How should a coder report a patient with multiple chronic conditions seen for a routine follow-up?'
'The coder should list the diagnosis codes in order of importance, starting with the primary reason for the visit. Each chronic condition should be coded separately unless a combination code is available. If the visit is primarily for managing diabetes with hypertension, the correct codes would be E11.9 (Type 2 diabetes mellitus without complications) and I10 (Essential hypertension).'

'What is the purpose of Z codes in ICD-10-CM?'
'Z codes are used for encounters that do not involve an active disease but instead relate to a patient's medical history, screening, vaccinations, follow-up care, or personal and social factors affecting health. For example, Z12.11 (Encounter for screening for malignant neoplasm of colon) is used for routine colon cancer screening.'

'How should a coder report a patient who presents for a well-woman exam?'
'A well-woman exam is coded with Z01.419 (Encounter for gynecological examination without abnormal findings) or Z01.411 (Encounter for gynecological examination with abnormal findings) if any abnormalities are detected.'

'What ICD-10-CM code should be used for an annual physical exam without any abnormal findings?'
'The correct code for an annual general health check-up without abnormal findings is Z00.00 (Encounter for general adult medical examination without abnormal findings). If abnormalities are found, Z00.01 should be used instead.'

'How should a coder report a patient who refuses a recommended vaccination?'
'If a patient refuses a vaccination, a Z code should be assigned to indicate this. The correct code is Z28.2 (Immunization not carried out because of patient decision for unspecified reason), or a more specific code such as Z28.0 (Immunization not carried out due to contraindication).'

'Why is it important to include an external cause code when reporting an injury?'
'External cause codes provide additional information on how an injury occurred, where it occurred, and whether it was intentional or accidental. These codes help with epidemiological tracking and legal documentation. For example, a patient who suffered a fractured wrist after slipping on ice should have both the injury code (S62.5XXA – Fracture of distal radius) and an external cause code (W00.0XXA – Fall due to ice and snow, initial encounter).'

'When coding fractures, what does the seventh character represent?'
'The seventh character in fracture coding provides details about the stage of treatment:'

- "A" – Initial encounter for fracture treatment'
- "D" – Subsequent encounter for healing fracture'
- "S" – Sequela, meaning the patient is being treated for complications from the previous fracture'

'What is the correct way to code a burn injury?'
'Burns are coded based on their depth (first, second, or third degree), the affected body area, and the extent of total body surface involved. A patient with second-degree burns on the right forearm and left hand would be coded with:'

- 'T22.211A (Second-degree burn of right forearm, initial encounter)'
- 'T23.202A (Second-degree burn of left hand, initial encounter)'

'How should a coder report a patient with a sprained ankle from a fall at home?'
'The primary diagnosis should be the injury code (S93.401A – Sprain of unspecified ligament of right ankle, initial encounter). The external cause code (W19.XXXA – Unspecified fall, initial encounter) and place of occurrence code (Y92.009 – Unspecified place in house) should also be included.'

'What is the proper way to code a patient returning for a follow-up visit after a broken femur?'
'If the patient is healing normally, the coder should use the appropriate fracture code with the seventh character "D" (subsequent encounter). For example, S72.001D (Fracture of unspecified part of femur, subsequent encounter for closed fracture).'

'How should hypertension with heart failure be coded?'
'Instead of using separate codes, a combination code should be assigned. The correct code is I11.0 (Hypertensive heart disease with heart failure). If the type of heart failure is documented, an additional code such as I50.22 (Chronic systolic heart failure) should be included.'

'What is the correct way to code a patient with both asthma and COPD?'
'If both asthma and COPD are documented, a combination code should be used instead of separate codes. The correct code is J44.9 (Chronic obstructive pulmonary disease, unspecified), along with a more specific asthma code if needed.'

'When coding diabetes with complications, what must be considered?'
'ICD-10-CM provides combination codes for diabetes with complications. The coder should ensure that the correct type of diabetes (Type 1 or Type 2) and all complications are documented. For example, E11.65 (Type 2 diabetes mellitus with hyperglycemia) is used if the patient has high blood sugar readings.'

'How is dementia with behavioral disturbances coded?'
'Dementia should be coded with both the primary condition and any associated behaviors. The correct code is F03.91 (Unspecified dementia with behavioral disturbance). If the dementia type is known (e.g., Alzheimer's), a more specific code should be used.'

'What is the correct way to code a stroke with residual left-sided weakness?'
'The primary code should indicate the history of the stroke, such as I69.354 (Hemiplegia and hemiparesis following cerebral infarction affecting left non-dominant side). Additional codes should be assigned for any ongoing treatments or complications.'

'What ICD-10-CM category is used for pregnancy-related conditions?'
'Pregnancy-related conditions are coded using Chapter 15 (O00-O9A) codes. These codes take sequencing priority over other diagnoses unless the reason for the visit is unrelated to pregnancy.'

'How should a coder report a patient with gestational diabetes treated with insulin?'
'The correct code is O24.414 (Gestational diabetes mellitus in pregnancy, insulin-controlled). The use of insulin should be documented and does not require an additional code.'

'How should a routine newborn checkup be coded?'
'A routine newborn checkup should be coded using Z00.110 (Health examination for newborn under 8 days old) or Z00.111 (Health examination for newborn 8 to 28 days old).'

'What is the correct way to report a mammogram screening for a woman with no symptoms?'
'If the patient has no symptoms, the correct code is Z12.31 (Encounter for screening mammogram for malignant neoplasm of breast). If a patient has a prior history of breast cancer, Z85.3 (Personal history of malignant neoplasm of breast) should also be included.'

'What is the correct way to code a patient who has completed chemotherapy and is in remission?'
'If the cancer is in remission, the appropriate ICD-10-CM code should be from category Z85 (Personal history of malignant neoplasm). If the remission status is not specified, the coder may need to clarify with the provider.'

'How should a coder report a patient seen for preoperative clearance before surgery?'
'The correct code for a preoperative clearance visit depends on the reason for the clearance. A general preoperative evaluation is coded with Z01.818 (Encounter for other preprocedural examination). An additional code for the condition requiring surgery should also be reported.'

'What is the correct way to code a patient receiving palliative care?'
'If a patient is receiving palliative or hospice care, the correct ICD-10-CM code is Z51.5 (Encounter for palliative care). This code should be listed along with any primary diagnosis responsible for the patient's need for palliative care.'

'How should a coder report a patient who has an allergy to penicillin?'
'Drug allergies are coded using Z88.0 (Allergy status to penicillin). This is important for tracking patient safety and preventing medication errors.'

'What is the correct ICD-10-CM code for a patient undergoing a routine eye exam with no abnormalities?'
'A routine eye exam with no issues is coded as Z01.00 (Encounter for examination of eyes and vision without abnormal findings). If an abnormal finding is discovered, Z01.01 should be used instead.'

'When should a coder use an unspecified code?'
'Unspecified codes should only be used when the provider's documentation does not provide enough detail for a more specific diagnosis. They should be avoided if detailed information is available.'

'How should a coder report a motor vehicle accident with multiple injuries?'
'The coder should list the primary injury first, followed by additional injuries and an external cause code for the accident. A code from V43-V49 (Occupant of car injured in transport accident) should be included to describe the circumstances of the crash.'

'What code should be used for an initial visit for a dog bite to the left hand?'
'The correct codes would be S61.452A (Open bite of left hand, initial encounter) along with W54.0XXA (Bitten by dog, initial encounter). The injury code should always be listed first, followed by the external cause code.'

'How should a coder report a fall from a wheelchair resulting in a fractured hip?'
'The correct coding sequence should include the primary injury (fractured hip), followed by an external cause code such as W05.0XXA (Fall from wheelchair, initial encounter) and a place of occurrence code (Y92.22, Home as place of occurrence).'

'What is the correct way to report an old traumatic brain injury with cognitive deficits?'
'A past traumatic brain injury with lasting cognitive effects is coded using S06.2X9S (Diffuse traumatic brain injury with sequela) along with an additional code from F07.81 (Postconcussional syndrome) or other codes to reflect specific cognitive deficits.'

'How should a coder report a patient with burns covering 30% of the total body surface area?'
'Burn coding requires documentation of the severity, location, and total body surface area affected. The correct code for total body surface area involvement is T31.30 (Burn involving 30-39% of body surface). Additional codes for the depth and location of each burn site should also be assigned.'

'What is the correct way to code a patient with COPD and chronic respiratory failure?'
'The primary code should be J44.9 (Chronic obstructive pulmonary disease, unspecified), followed by J96.10 (Chronic respiratory failure, unspecified whether hypoxia or hypercapnia).'

'How should a coder report a patient with anemia due to chemotherapy?'
'The correct coding sequence is D64.81 (Anemia due to antineoplastic chemotherapy) followed by Z51.11 (Encounter for antineoplastic chemotherapy).'

'What is the correct way to code a patient with end-stage renal disease requiring dialysis?'
'End-stage renal disease should be reported using N18.6 (End-stage renal disease), along with Z99.2 (Dependence on renal dialysis) to indicate ongoing treatment.'

'How should a coder report a patient with heart failure and chronic kidney disease stage 4 due to hypertension?'
'A combination code should be used for hypertensive heart and kidney disease. The correct coding sequence is I13.10 (Hypertensive heart and chronic kidney disease without heart failure, with stage 1-4 CKD) and N18.4 (Chronic kidney disease, stage 4).'

'What code should be assigned for a patient with obesity due to excessive calorie intake?'
'The correct code is E66.0 (Obesity due to excess calories). If the patient has morbid obesity, E66.01 should be used instead.'

'How should a coder report a patient seen for prenatal care with no complications?'
'A routine prenatal visit without complications is coded with Z34.90 (Encounter for supervision of normal pregnancy, unspecified trimester). If the trimester is documented, a more specific code such as Z34.81 (Supervision of normal first pregnancy, first trimester) should be used.'

'What ICD-10-CM code is used for a newborn diagnosed with neonatal jaundice?'
'Neonatal jaundice is coded as P59.9 (Neonatal jaundice, unspecified). If the type of jaundice is known, a more specific code should be used.'

'How should a coder report a woman undergoing screening for cervical cancer?'
'The correct code is Z12.4 (Encounter for screening for malignant neoplasm of cervix). If the screening is done as part of a routine well-woman exam, Z01.419 should also be assigned.'

'How should a coder report a patient with a history of gestational diabetes now undergoing postpartum follow-up?'
'A patient with a history of gestational diabetes should be coded with Z86.32 (Personal history of gestational diabetes).'

'What is the correct way to code a newborn who is small for gestational age?'
'Small for gestational age is coded as P05.10 (Newborn small for gestational age, unspecified weeks of gestation). If the exact gestational weeks are documented, a more specific code such as P05.18 (Small for gestational age, 37 or more completed weeks) should be used.'

'How should a coder report a patient who presents with a confirmed case of influenza A?'
'The correct code for a confirmed case of influenza A is J10.1 (Influenza due to identified influenza A virus with other respiratory manifestations). If the patient also has pneumonia, an additional code such as J12.89 (Other viral pneumonia) should be assigned.'

'What is the correct way to code a patient with acute appendicitis with perforation?'
'The appropriate code for acute appendicitis with perforation is K35.2 (Acute appendicitis with generalized peritonitis). If the patient underwent an appendectomy, a procedure code from ICD-10-PCS should also be assigned.'

'How should a coder report a patient diagnosed with primary open-angle glaucoma in both eyes?'
'The correct code for bilateral primary open-angle glaucoma is H40.11X3 (Primary open-angle glaucoma, bilateral, severe stage). The last digit should reflect the documented stage of the condition.'

'What is the correct way to code a patient who has an allergic reaction to peanuts?'
'The correct ICD-10-CM code for an allergic reaction to peanuts is T78.01XA (Anaphylactic reaction due to peanuts, initial encounter). If the reaction is not anaphylactic, a more appropriate code such as Z91.010 (Allergy to peanuts) should be used.'

'How should a coder report a patient with chronic migraines that include aura?'
'The correct code for chronic migraines with aura is G43.109 (Chronic migraine without aura, not intractable). If the migraines are intractable, a different subcategory should be selected to reflect the severity and resistance to treatment.'

'What is the correct way to code a patient with an inguinal hernia that is obstructed but not gangrenous?'
'The correct ICD-10-CM code for an obstructed but non-gangrenous inguinal hernia is K40.30 (Bilateral inguinal hernia, with obstruction, without gangrene). If the hernia was repaired surgically, a procedure code should be included.'

'How should a coder report a patient diagnosed with carpal tunnel syndrome in both wrists?'
'The correct code for bilateral carpal tunnel syndrome is G56.03 (Carpal tunnel syndrome, bilateral upper limbs). If the condition requires surgical correction, an ICD-10-PCS procedure code should also be assigned.'

'What is the correct way to code a patient diagnosed with stage 2 pressure ulcer of the sacrum?'
'The correct code for a stage 2 pressure ulcer of the sacrum is L89.152 (Pressure ulcer of sacral region, stage 2). The last digit in the code must correspond to the severity of the ulcer, ranging from stage 1 to stage 4 or unstageable.'

'How should a coder report a patient undergoing follow-up after a kidney transplant due to chronic kidney disease?'
'The correct primary code is Z48.22 (Encounter for aftercare following kidney transplant). An additional code such as N18.9 (Chronic kidney disease, unspecified) should be used if the transplanted kidney is affected by any condition.'

'What is the correct way to code a patient diagnosed with iron deficiency anemia secondary to chronic blood loss?'
'The correct ICD-10-CM code for iron deficiency anemia due to chronic blood loss is D50.0 (Iron deficiency anemia secondary to blood loss [chronic]). The cause of the blood loss should also be documented and coded if known.'

'How should a coder report a patient with alcoholic cirrhosis of the liver with ascites?'
'The correct ICD-10-CM code is K70.31 (Alcoholic cirrhosis of liver with ascites). If complications such as hepatic encephalopathy are present, additional codes should be assigned.'

'What is the correct way to code a patient with schizophrenia, paranoid type, currently in exacerbation?'
'The correct code for paranoid schizophrenia in exacerbation is F20.0 (Paranoid schizophrenia). If the documentation specifies acute exacerbation, the coder should ensure the correct severity level is reported.'

'How should a coder report a patient diagnosed with hyperthyroidism with thyrotoxic crisis?'
'The correct ICD-10-CM code for hyperthyroidism with a thyrotoxic crisis is E05.01 (Thyrotoxicosis with thyroid storm). This code captures both the underlying thyroid condition and the life-threatening crisis.'

'What is the correct way to code a patient diagnosed with Bell's palsy?'
'The correct ICD-10-CM code for Bell's palsy is G51.0 (Bell's palsy). If the condition resolves, it does not require follow-up coding unless complications persist.'

'How should a coder report a newborn diagnosed with neonatal hypoglycemia?'
'The correct ICD-10-CM code for neonatal hypoglycemia is P70.4 (Neonatal hypoglycemia). If the hypoglycemia is related to maternal diabetes, a secondary code such as P70.1 (Neonatal hypoglycemia due to maternal diabetes) should also be assigned.'

'What is the correct way to code a patient diagnosed with chronic venous insufficiency in both lower extremities?'
'The correct ICD-10-CM code for chronic venous insufficiency in both lower extremities is I87.2 (Chronic venous hypertension [venous insufficiency] [peripheral venous incompetence]). If there is an associated ulcer, additional codes should be included.'

'How should a coder report a patient presenting with acute pyelonephritis?'
'The correct ICD-10-CM code for acute pyelonephritis is N10 (Acute pyelonephritis). If the pyelonephritis is due to an identified bacterial organism, an additional code from B95-B97 should be used to specify the responsible pathogen.'

'What is the correct way to code a patient diagnosed with chronic pancreatitis due to alcohol use?'
'The correct ICD-10-CM code for chronic pancreatitis due to alcohol use is K86.0 (Alcohol-induced chronic pancreatitis). If the patient has a history of alcoholism, F10.20 (Alcohol dependence, uncomplicated) should be assigned.'

'How should a coder report a patient diagnosed with obstructive sleep apnea requiring CPAP therapy?'
'The correct ICD-10-CM code for obstructive sleep apnea is G47.33 (Obstructive sleep apnea [adult] [pediatric]). If the patient is using CPAP therapy, it should be documented but does not require an additional diagnosis code.'

'How should a coder report a patient diagnosed with acute bronchitis due to Mycoplasma pneumoniae?'
'The correct ICD-10-CM code for acute bronchitis due to Mycoplasma pneumoniae is J20.0 (Acute bronchitis due to Mycoplasma pneumoniae). If the patient also has underlying chronic conditions such as COPD, an additional code for the pre-existing condition should be assigned.'

'What is the correct way to code a patient with persistent depressive disorder with intermittent major depressive episodes?'
'The correct ICD-10-CM code for this condition is F34.81 (Persistent depressive disorder with intermittent major depressive episodes). If the depressive episodes are documented as severe, additional coding may be required for more specificity.'

'How should a coder report a patient diagnosed with a gangrenous pressure ulcer of the left heel?'
'The correct ICD-10-CM code is L89.624 (Pressure ulcer of left heel, stage 4). If the provider documents gangrene, an additional code such as I96 (Gangrene, not elsewhere classified) should be used.'

'What is the correct way to code a patient diagnosed with ankylosing spondylitis?'
'The correct ICD-10-CM code for ankylosing spondylitis is M45.9 (Ankylosing spondylitis of unspecified site). If a specific region of the spine is affected, a more detailed code such as M45.4 (Ankylosing spondylitis of cervical region) should be used.'

'How should a coder report a patient diagnosed with polycystic ovarian syndrome (PCOS)?'
'The correct ICD-10-CM code for polycystic ovarian syndrome is E28.2 (Polycystic ovarian syndrome). If the patient has related conditions such as insulin resistance, an additional code may be needed.'

'What is the correct way to code a patient diagnosed with a retinal detachment with macular hole in the right eye?'
'The correct ICD-10-CM code is H33.051 (Retinal detachment with retinal break, right eye). If surgery is performed to repair the detachment, an additional ICD-10-PCS procedure code should be assigned.'

'How should a coder report a patient presenting with a Bartholin's gland abscess?'
'The correct ICD-10-CM code for a Bartholin's gland abscess is N75.0 (Abscess of Bartholin's gland). If the abscess requires drainage, a procedure code should also be assigned.'

'What is the correct way to code a patient with a traumatic pneumothorax following a rib fracture?'
'The correct ICD-10-CM code is S27.0XXA (Traumatic pneumothorax, initial encounter). An additional code for the rib fracture, such as S22.41XA (Fracture of one rib, initial encounter), should also be assigned.'

'How should a coder report a patient diagnosed with lumbosacral radiculopathy?'
'The correct ICD-10-CM code for lumbosacral radiculopathy is M54.17 (Radiculopathy, lumbosacral region). If the radiculopathy is due to a herniated disc, a more specific code should be used.'

'What is the correct way to code a patient diagnosed with non-ST elevation myocardial infarction (NSTEMI)?'
'The correct ICD-10-CM code for NSTEMI is I21.4 (Non-ST elevation myocardial infarction). If the provider documents a subsequent NSTEMI, I22.2 (Subsequent non-ST elevation myocardial infarction) should be used instead.'

'How should a coder report a patient with bacterial vaginosis?'
'The correct ICD-10-CM code for bacterial vaginosis is N76.0 (Acute vaginitis). If the provider specifies Gardnerella vaginalis as the causative organism, an additional code such as B96.89 (Other specified bacterial agents as the cause of diseases classified elsewhere) may be assigned.'

'What is the correct way to code a patient with a ruptured Achilles tendon?'
'The correct ICD-10-CM code for a ruptured Achilles tendon is S86.019A (Other injury of Achilles tendon, unspecified leg, initial encounter). If the provider specifies the laterality, a more detailed code such as S86.011A (Strain of right Achilles tendon, initial encounter) should be used.'

'How should a coder report a patient diagnosed with hereditary spherocytosis?'
'The correct ICD-10-CM code for hereditary spherocytosis is D58.0 (Hereditary spherocytosis). If the patient has an associated hemolytic crisis, additional coding should be considered.'

'What is the correct way to code a patient diagnosed with major neurocognitive disorder due to Alzheimer's disease?'
'The correct ICD-10-CM code for this condition is G30.9 (Alzheimer's disease, unspecified) along with F02.80 (Dementia in other diseases classified elsewhere without behavioral disturbance). If behavioral disturbances are present, F02.81 should be used instead.'

'How should a coder report a patient diagnosed with hidradenitis suppurativa?'
'The correct ICD-10-CM code for hidradenitis suppurativa is L73.2 (Hidradenitis suppurativa). If the condition affects multiple sites, additional codes may be necessary to specify the location.'

'What is the correct way to code a patient with acute cholecystitis with gallstones?'
'The correct ICD-10-CM code for acute cholecystitis with gallstones is K80.00 (Calculus of gallbladder with acute cholecystitis without obstruction). If obstruction is present, K80.01 should be used instead.'

'How should a coder report a patient with chronic fatigue syndrome?'
'The correct ICD-10-CM code for chronic fatigue syndrome is R53.82 (Chronic fatigue syndrome, unspecified). If the provider documents post-viral fatigue syndrome, a different code such as G93.3 (Postviral fatigue syndrome) should be assigned.'

'What is the correct way to code a patient with a benign meningioma of the brain?'
'The correct ICD-10-CM code for a benign meningioma of the brain is D32.0 (Benign neoplasm of cerebral meninges). If the meningioma is in a different part of the brain, a more specific code should be used.'

'How should a coder report a patient diagnosed with congenital hip dysplasia?'
'The correct ICD-10-CM code for congenital hip dysplasia is Q65.0 (Congenital dislocation of hip, unilateral). If both hips are affected, Q65.1 (Congenital dislocation of hip, bilateral) should be used instead.'

'What is the correct way to code a patient diagnosed with Zollinger-Ellison syndrome?'
'The correct ICD-10-CM code for Zollinger-Ellison syndrome is E16.4 (Zollinger-Ellison syndrome). If complications such as peptic ulcers are present, additional codes should be assigned to reflect those conditions.'

'How should a coder report a patient diagnosed with lead poisoning?'
'The correct ICD-10-CM code for lead poisoning is T56.0X1A (Toxic effect of lead and its compounds, accidental, initial encounter). If chronic exposure is documented, a different code should be used.'

'How should a coder report a patient diagnosed with serotonin syndrome due to medication interaction?'
'The correct ICD-10-CM code for serotonin syndrome is T43.95XA (Adverse effect of other psychotropic drugs, initial encounter). If the specific drug causing the reaction is known, an additional code from the T36-T50 series should be assigned.'

'What is the correct way to code a patient with a spontaneous pneumothorax?'
'The correct ICD-10-CM code for spontaneous pneumothorax is J93.11 (Primary spontaneous pneumothorax). If the pneumothorax is secondary to an underlying condition, a different code such as J93.12 (Secondary spontaneous pneumothorax) should be used.'

'How should a coder report a patient diagnosed with transient global amnesia?'
'The correct ICD-10-CM code for transient global amnesia is G45.4 (Transient global amnesia). If there is an associated condition, it should be coded separately.'

'What is the correct way to code a patient diagnosed with chronic anal fissure?'
'The correct ICD-10-CM code for chronic anal fissure is K60.2 (Chronic anal fissure). If the fissure is acute, K60.0 should be used instead.'

'How should a coder report a patient with spinal stenosis of the lumbar region with neurogenic claudication?'
'The correct ICD-10-CM code for spinal stenosis with neurogenic claudication is M48.062 (Spinal stenosis, lumbar region with neurogenic claudication). This code includes both the stenosis and the associated claudication, eliminating the need for separate coding.'

'What is the correct way to code a patient diagnosed with Gilbert's syndrome?'
'The correct ICD-10-CM code for Gilbert's syndrome is E80.4 (Gilbert syndrome). This condition is a benign liver disorder that does not typically require extensive medical treatment.'

'How should a coder report a patient presenting with drug-induced lupus erythematosus?'
'The correct ICD-10-CM code for drug-induced lupus is M32.0 (Drug-induced systemic lupus erythematosus). If the offending drug is identified, an additional code from the T36-T50 series should be assigned to specify the drug involved.'

'What is the correct way to code a patient diagnosed with postherpetic neuralgia?'
'The correct ICD-10-CM code for postherpetic neuralgia is B02.22 (Postherpetic neuralgia). If the patient has active herpes zoster, an additional code for the current herpes infection should be reported.'

'How should a coder report a patient with congenital hydrocephalus?'
'The correct ICD-10-CM code for congenital hydrocephalus is Q03.9 (Congenital hydrocephalus, unspecified). If the hydrocephalus is due to a specific congenital cause, a more detailed code should be used.'

'What is the correct way to code a patient diagnosed with serotonin deficiency syndrome?'
'The correct ICD-10-CM code for serotonin deficiency syndrome is E63.8 (Other specified nutritional deficiencies). Since there is no specific code for serotonin deficiency, this code best describes the condition.'

'How should a coder report a patient diagnosed with tibial stress fracture due to overuse?'
'The correct ICD-10-CM code for a tibial stress fracture is M84.364A (Stress fracture, right tibia, initial encounter). If the opposite leg is affected, M84.365A should be used instead.'

'What is the correct way to code a patient with Lyme disease?'
'The correct ICD-10-CM code for Lyme disease is A69.20 (Lyme disease, unspecified). If the patient has neurological or joint manifestations, additional codes should be assigned to reflect those complications.'

'How should a coder report a patient diagnosed with Klinefelter syndrome?'
'The correct ICD-10-CM code for Klinefelter syndrome is Q98.4 (Klinefelter syndrome, unspecified). If a specific karyotype is documented, a more detailed code from the Q98 category should be used.'

'What is the correct way to code a patient presenting with hypovolemic shock?'
'The correct ICD-10-CM code for hypovolemic shock is R57.1 (Hypovolemic shock). If the shock is due to blood loss, an additional code such as D62 (Acute posthemorrhagic anemia) should be assigned.'

'How should a coder report a patient diagnosed with chronic Achilles tendinitis in the right leg?'
'The correct ICD-10-CM code for chronic Achilles tendinitis of the right leg is M76.61 (Achilles tendinitis, right leg). If the left leg is affected, M76.62 should be used instead.'

'What is the correct way to code a patient diagnosed with restless leg syndrome?'
'The correct ICD-10-CM code for restless leg syndrome is G25.81 (Restless legs syndrome). If the condition is secondary to another disorder, that disorder should also be coded.'

'How should a coder report a patient diagnosed with post-concussion syndrome?'
'The correct ICD-10-CM code for post-concussion syndrome is F07.81 (Postconcussional syndrome). If the initial concussion diagnosis is still being treated, an additional code from the S06 category should be assigned.'

'What is the correct way to code a patient diagnosed with seborrheic keratosis?'
'The correct ICD-10-CM code for seborrheic keratosis is L82.0 (Inflamed seborrheic keratosis). If the condition is not inflamed, L82.1 should be used instead.'

'How should a coder report a patient diagnosed with psoriatic arthritis?'
'The correct ICD-10-CM code for psoriatic arthritis is L40.50 (Arthropathic psoriasis, unspecified). If the type of psoriatic arthritis is specified, a more detailed code should be used.'

'What is the correct way to code a patient presenting with a colles fracture?'
'The correct ICD-10-CM code for a Colles fracture is S52.531A (Colles' fracture of right radius, initial encounter). If the left radius is affected, S52.532A should be used instead.'

'How should a coder report a patient diagnosed with a prolapsed rectum?'
'The correct ICD-10-CM code for a prolapsed rectum is K62.3 (Rectal prolapse). If the condition is recurrent or postoperative, an additional code should be considered.'

'What is the correct way to code a patient diagnosed with swimmer's ear?'
'The correct ICD-10-CM code for swimmer's ear is H60.33 (Swimmer's ear, bilateral). If the infection is only in one ear, H60.31 (right ear) or H60.32 (left ear) should be used.'

'How should a coder report a patient diagnosed with chronic Epstein-Barr virus infection?'
'The correct ICD-10-CM code for chronic Epstein-Barr virus infection is B27.10 (Chronic infectious mononucleosis, unspecified). If the condition is associated with another complication, additional codes should be assigned.'

'What is the correct way to code a patient diagnosed with mild cognitive impairment?'
'The correct ICD-10-CM code for mild cognitive impairment is G31.84 (Mild cognitive impairment, so stated). If the patient has a history of a related neurological condition, that should also be coded.'

'How should a coder report a patient diagnosed with chronic vestibular migraine?'
'The correct ICD-10-CM code for a vestibular migraine is G43.D0 (Vestibular migraine, not intractable, without status migrainosus). If the migraine is intractable, a different seventh character should be assigned.'

'What is the correct way to code a patient with a Baker's cyst in the left knee?'
'The correct ICD-10-CM code for a Baker's cyst in the left knee is M71.22 (Other bursitis of left knee). If the condition is associated with osteoarthritis, an additional code should be included.'

'How should a coder report a patient diagnosed with eosinophilic esophagitis?'
'The correct ICD-10-CM code for eosinophilic esophagitis is K20.0 (Eosinophilic esophagitis). If the patient has associated gastroesophageal reflux disease (GERD), it should be coded separately.'

'What is the correct way to code a patient diagnosed with an Achilles tendon rupture that has not been treated?'
'The correct ICD-10-CM code for an old, untreated Achilles tendon rupture is M66.37 (Spontaneous rupture of other tendons, ankle and foot). If the rupture is acute, an S-code from the injury chapter should be used instead.'

'How should a coder report a patient presenting with reactive arthritis following a gastrointestinal infection?'
'The correct ICD-10-CM code for reactive arthritis is M02.9 (Reactive arthropathy, unspecified). If the specific infection that triggered the arthritis is known, an additional code should be used to specify the infectious agent.'

'What is the correct way to code a patient diagnosed with femoroacetabular impingement syndrome (FAI)?'
'The correct ICD-10-CM code for femoroacetabular impingement syndrome is M24.851 (Femoroacetabular impingement, right hip). If the left hip is affected, M24.852 should be assigned instead.'

'How should a coder report a patient diagnosed with Pott's disease (tuberculosis of the spine)?'
'The correct ICD-10-CM code for Pott's disease is A18.01 (Tuberculosis of spine). If there are neurological complications, additional codes may be required.'

'What is the correct way to code a patient diagnosed with trigeminal neuralgia?'
'The correct ICD-10-CM code for trigeminal neuralgia is G50.0 (Trigeminal neuralgia). If the condition is secondary to another disorder, that should also be coded.'

'How should a coder report a patient diagnosed with exertional rhabdomyolysis?'
'The correct ICD-10-CM code for exertional rhabdomyolysis is M62.82 (Rhabdomyolysis). If the patient also has acute kidney injury due to rhabdomyolysis, N17.9 (Acute kidney failure, unspecified) should be assigned.'

'What is the correct way to code a patient diagnosed with adhesive capsulitis of the right shoulder?'
'The correct ICD-10-CM code for adhesive capsulitis of the right shoulder is M75.01 (Adhesive capsulitis of right shoulder). If the left shoulder is affected, M75.02 should be used instead.'

'How should a coder report a patient presenting with recurrent small bowel obstruction?'
'The correct ICD-10-CM code for recurrent small bowel obstruction is K56.50 (Intestinal adhesions with obstruction, unspecified). If the obstruction is due to postoperative adhesions, a more specific code from K56.51 should be used.'

'What is the correct way to code a patient diagnosed with thoracic outlet syndrome?'
'The correct ICD-10-CM code for thoracic outlet syndrome is G54.0 (Brachial plexus disorders). If the provider specifies the type of thoracic outlet syndrome (neurogenic, arterial, venous), additional codes should be used.'

'How should a coder report a patient diagnosed with a hypercoagulable state due to an inherited clotting disorder?'
'The correct ICD-10-CM code for an inherited hypercoagulable state is D68.59 (Other primary thrombophilia). If the provider specifies Factor V Leiden mutation, D68.51 should be used instead.'

'What is the correct way to code a patient diagnosed with an acute meniscus tear of the left knee?'
'The correct ICD-10-CM code for an acute medial meniscus tear of the left knee is S83.242A (Tear of medial meniscus, current injury, left knee, initial encounter). If it is a chronic tear, M23.202 should be used.'

'How should a coder report a patient diagnosed with post-traumatic stress disorder (PTSD) with nightmares and flashbacks?'
'The correct ICD-10-CM code for PTSD is F43.10 (Post-traumatic stress disorder, unspecified). If the PTSD is specified as chronic or acute, a more detailed code should be selected.'

'What is the correct way to code a patient with an impacted cerumen in both ears?'
'The correct ICD-10-CM code for impacted cerumen in both ears is H61.23 (Impacted cerumen, bilateral). If only one ear is affected, H61.21 (right ear) or H61.22 (left ear) should be used.'

'How should a coder report a patient diagnosed with a splenic infarction?'
'The correct ICD-10-CM code for a splenic infarction is D73.5 (Infarction of spleen). If the condition is due to an underlying hypercoagulable disorder, an additional code should be assigned.'

'What is the correct way to code a patient diagnosed with nummular eczema?'
'The correct ICD-10-CM code for nummular eczema is L30.0 (Nummular dermatitis). If the condition is chronic, it should still be reported under the same code.'

'How should a coder report a patient diagnosed with an intrahepatic cholangiocarcinoma?'
'The correct ICD-10-CM code for an intrahepatic cholangiocarcinoma is C22.1 (Intrahepatic bile duct carcinoma). If the condition has metastasized, additional codes should be included for secondary malignancies.'

'How should a coder report a patient diagnosed with thoracic aortic aneurysm without rupture?'
'The correct ICD-10-CM code for a thoracic aortic aneurysm without rupture is I71.2 (Thoracic aortic aneurysm, without rupture). If the aneurysm is ruptured, I71.1 should be used instead.'

'What is the correct way to code a patient diagnosed with subclinical hypothyroidism?'
'The correct ICD-10-CM code for subclinical hypothyroidism is E02 (Subclinical iodine-deficiency hypothyroidism). If the provider documents primary hypothyroidism, E03.9 should be used instead.'

'How should a coder report a patient diagnosed with acute gastritis with bleeding?'
'The correct ICD-10-CM code for acute gastritis with bleeding is K29.01 (Acute gastritis with bleeding). If chronic gastritis is also present, an additional code from K29.5- should be assigned.'

'What is the correct way to code a patient diagnosed with a retinal artery occlusion of the left eye?'
'The correct ICD-10-CM code for a retinal artery occlusion of the left eye is H34.11 (Central retinal artery occlusion, left eye). If the occlusion is branch-related, a different H34 code should be used.'

'How should a coder report a patient diagnosed with neonatal abstinence syndrome due to maternal opioid use?'
'The correct ICD-10-CM code for neonatal abstinence syndrome due to maternal opioid use is P96.1 (Neonatal withdrawal symptoms from maternal use of drugs of addiction). If the specific drug is documented, an additional code should be assigned.'

'What is the correct way to code a patient diagnosed with a scaphoid fracture in the right wrist?'
'The correct ICD-10-CM code for a right wrist scaphoid fracture is S62.011A (Fracture of scaphoid bone of right wrist, initial encounter). If the left wrist is affected, S62.012A should be used instead.'

'How should a coder report a patient diagnosed with viral conjunctivitis?'
'The correct ICD-10-CM code for viral conjunctivitis is B30.9 (Viral conjunctivitis, unspecified). If the cause is known, such as adenovirus, a more specific B30 code should be assigned.'

'What is the correct way to code a patient diagnosed with a Bartholin's gland cyst?'
'The correct ICD-10-CM code for a Bartholin's gland cyst is N75.1 (Cyst of Bartholin's gland). If the cyst is infected or abscessed, N75.0 should be used instead.'

'How should a coder report a patient diagnosed with alcoholic gastritis?'
'The correct ICD-10-CM code for alcoholic gastritis is K29.20 (Alcoholic gastritis without bleeding). If there is active bleeding, K29.21 should be used instead.'

'What is the correct way to code a patient diagnosed with osteomyelitis of the left tibia?'
'The correct ICD-10-CM code for osteomyelitis of the left tibia depends on the type. For acute hematogenous osteomyelitis, M86.162 (Acute hematogenous osteomyelitis, left tibia and fibula) should be used. If the osteomyelitis is chronic, a different M86 code should be selected.'

'How should a coder report a patient diagnosed with a congenital diaphragmatic hernia?'
'The correct ICD-10-CM code for a congenital diaphragmatic hernia is Q79.0 (Congenital diaphragmatic hernia). If there are associated respiratory complications, additional codes should be assigned.'

'What is the correct way to code a patient diagnosed with chronic pelvic inflammatory disease?'
'The correct ICD-10-CM code for chronic pelvic inflammatory disease is N73.6 (Chronic pelvic peritonitis). If the condition is acute, N73.2 should be used instead.'

'How should a coder report a patient diagnosed with toxic shock syndrome?'
'The correct ICD-10-CM code for toxic shock syndrome is A48.3 (Toxic shock syndrome). If the condition is due to a specific bacterial infection, an additional code should be assigned to specify the organism.'

'What is the correct way to code a patient diagnosed with an umbilical hernia with obstruction but no gangrene?'
'The correct ICD-10-CM code for an umbilical hernia with obstruction but no gangrene is K42.0 (Umbilical hernia with obstruction, without gangrene). If gangrene is present, K42.1 should be used instead.'

'How should a coder report a patient diagnosed with cellulitis of the left lower leg?'
'The correct ICD-10-CM code for cellulitis of the left lower leg is L03.116 (Cellulitis of left lower limb). If there is an associated abscess, a combination code such as L03.119 should be used instead.'

'What is the correct way to code a patient diagnosed with a congenital adrenal hyperplasia?'
'The correct ICD-10-CM code for congenital adrenal hyperplasia is E25.0 (Congenital adrenal hyperplasia). If the type is specified, a more detailed code should be selected.'

'How should a coder report a patient diagnosed with gestational hypertension without proteinuria in the third trimester?'
'The correct ICD-10-CM code for gestational hypertension without significant proteinuria in the third trimester is O13.3 (Gestational hypertension without significant proteinuria, third trimester). If proteinuria is present, preeclampsia should be considered and coded accordingly.'

'What is the correct way to code a patient diagnosed with Munchausen syndrome?'
'The correct ICD-10-CM code for Munchausen syndrome is F68.1 (Factitious disorder imposed on self). If the condition involves the falsification of illness in another person, F68.10 should be used instead.'

'How should a coder report a patient diagnosed with essential tremor?'
'The correct ICD-10-CM code for essential tremor is G25.0 (Essential tremor). If the tremor is due to another neurological disorder, an additional code should be assigned to specify the underlying cause.'

PRACTICE TEST

1. 'Which of the following codes is used for a patient diagnosed with benign prostatic hyperplasia with lower urinary tract symptoms?
a) N40.0
b) N40.1
c) N41.9
d) N13.8

2. 'A patient is diagnosed with chronic kidney disease stage 3. What is the correct ICD-10-CM **code?**
a) N18.3
b) N18.4
c) N18.9
d) N18.1

3. 'Which seventh character should be used for an initial encounter for a displaced tibial fracture?
a) A
b) D
c) S
d) C

4. 'What is the correct ICD-10-CM **code for a patient diagnosed with tension-type headache?**
a) G44.209
b) G43.909
c) R51.9
d) G44.001

5. 'Which ICD-10-CM **code should be assigned for a patient diagnosed with type 2 diabetes mellitus with hyperglycemia?**
a) E11.9
b) E11.65
c) E11.22
d) E11.40

6. 'A patient presents with a confirmed case of influenza A with pneumonia. What is the correct code assignment?
a) J10.1
b) J09.X2
c) J11.00
d) J10.00

7. 'Which of the following ICD-10-CM **codes represents a patient with acute myocardial infarction of the anterior wall?**
a) I21.01
b) I21.3
c) I21.4
d) I22.1

8. 'What is the correct ICD-10-CM **code for a patient diagnosed with chronic viral hepatitis C?**
a) B18.2
b) B17.10
c) B19.20
d) B18.0

9. 'Which of the following codes should be used for a patient with secondary hypertension?
a) I15.9
b) I10
c) I12.9
d) I13.0

10. 'A newborn is diagnosed with transient tachypnea. What is the correct ICD-10-CM **code?**
a) P22.1
b) P22.0
c) P28.5
d) P27.1

11. 'Which ICD-10-CM **code should be assigned for a patient with gastroesophageal reflux disease with esophagitis?**
a) K21.9
b) K21.0
c) K20.8
d) K22.70

12. 'A patient is diagnosed with acute cholecystitis with gallstones and obstruction. What is the correct ICD-10-CM **code?**
a) K80.00
b) K80.10
c) K80.12
d) K80.01

13. 'What is the correct ICD-10-CM **code for a patient with viral meningitis caused by enterovirus?**
a) A87.0
b) A87.8
c) A87.9
d) B34.1

14. 'Which of the following ICD-10-CM **codes is used for a patient diagnosed with postpartum hemorrhage?**
a) O72.0
b) O72.1
c) O72.2
d) O71.9

15. 'Which ICD-10-CM **code should be assigned for a patient diagnosed with schizophrenia, paranoid type?**
a) F20.0
b) F20.1
c) F20.2
d) F20.9

16. 'What is the correct ICD-10-CM code for a patient diagnosed with mild nonproliferative diabetic retinopathy with macular edema?
a) E11.329
b) E11.321
c) E11.311
d) E11.331

17. 'Which of the following ICD-10-CM codes represents a patient with chronic gout with tophi in the left ankle?
a) M10.072
b) M1A.0720
c) M10.271
d) M1A.2710

18. 'A patient is diagnosed with interstitial cystitis without hematuria. What is the correct ICD-10-CM code?
a) N30.10
b) N30.11
c) N32.89
d) N30.00

19. 'Which ICD-10-CM code is used for a patient diagnosed with multiple sclerosis?
a) G35
b) G37.9
c) G36.0
d) G37.8

20. 'What is the correct ICD-10-CM code for a patient diagnosed with Bell's palsy?
a) G51.0
b) G51.1
c) G50.1
d) G52.0

21. 'Which ICD-10-CM code should be assigned for a patient with acute pancreatitis without necrosis or infection?
a) K85.0
b) K85.9
c) K85.1
d) K85.3

22. 'A patient is diagnosed with primary osteoporosis with a current pathological fracture of the vertebra. What is the correct ICD-10-CM code?
a) M80.08XA
b) M81.0
c) M80.00XA
d) M80.80XA

23. 'Which of the following ICD-10-CM codes represents a patient diagnosed with moderate persistent asthma with status asthmaticus?
a) J45.40
b) J45.42
c) J45.50
d) J45.51

24. 'A patient is diagnosed with secondary Parkinsonism due to another medical condition. What is the correct ICD-10-CM code?
a) G21.8
b) G20
c) G21.3
d) G21.0

25. 'Which ICD-10-CM code should be assigned for a patient diagnosed with a traumatic subdural hemorrhage with loss of consciousness greater than 24 hours?
a) S06.5X5A
b) S06.5X9A
c) S06.5X4A
d) S06.5X6A

26. 'A patient presents with a left-sided hemiplegia due to an old cerebral infarction. What is the correct ICD-10-CM code?
a) I69.354
b) I69.351
c) I69.341
d) I69.342

27. 'Which ICD-10-CM code is used for a patient diagnosed with hypokalemia?
a) E87.6
b) E87.8
c) E87.2
d) E87.1

28. 'What is the correct ICD-10-CM code for a patient diagnosed with sepsis due to E. coli?
a) A41.51
b) A41.4
c) A41.2
d) A41.3

29. 'A patient is diagnosed with osteoarthritis of the right hip. What is the correct ICD-10-CM code?
a) M16.11
b) M16.12
c) M16.0
d) M16.9

30. 'A 45-year-old female presents with severe right lower quadrant pain. Imaging confirms acute appendicitis with perforation but no abscess. What is the correct ICD-10-CM code?
a) K35.20
b) K35.32
c) K35.80
d) K36

31. 'A 60-year-old male is diagnosed with hypertensive chronic kidney disease, stage 4. What is the correct code assignment?
a) I12.0, N18.4
b) I12.9, N18.4
c) I13.10, N18.4
d) I10, N18.4

32. 'A 32-year-old pregnant woman at 30 weeks gestation is diagnosed with pre-eclampsia with severe features. What is the correct ICD-10-CM **code?**
a) O14.90
b) O14.12
c) O14.10
d) O14.02

33. 'A 55-year-old male presents with unstable angina. His medical history includes hypertension and type 2 diabetes. What is the correct ICD-10-CM **code for the angina?**
a) I20.0
b) I20.1
c) I20.9
d) I25.119

34. 'A newborn is diagnosed with meconium aspiration syndrome and respiratory distress. What is the correct ICD-10-CM **code?**
a) P24.00
b) P24.30
c) P22.9
d) P22.1

35. 'A 67-year-old male presents with acute systolic heart failure. What is the correct ICD-10-CM **code?**
a) I50.1
b) I50.21
c) I50.22
d) I50.23

36. 'A patient with end-stage renal disease is on dialysis. What is the correct ICD-10-CM **code to indicate dialysis dependence?**
a) N18.6
b) Z99.2
c) N18.9
d) Z91.15

37. 'A 48-year-old male presents with alcohol dependence with intoxication and withdrawal. What is the correct ICD-10-CM **code?**
a) F10.129
b) F10.231
c) F10.239
d) F10.921

38. 'A 29-year-old female is diagnosed with gestational diabetes, diet controlled, in her second trimester. What is the correct ICD-10-CM **code?**
a) O24.419
b) O24.414
c) O24.012
d) O24.311

39. 'A 70-year-old female presents with an open fracture of the right femur due to a fall. What seventh character should be assigned for the initial encounter?
a) A
b) D
c) S
d) B

40. 'A 50-year-old male presents with left-sided Bell's palsy. What is the correct ICD-10-CM code?
a) G50.0
b) G51.0
c) G52.1
d) G54.2

41. 'A 35-year-old female presents with generalized anxiety disorder. What is the correct ICD-10-CM code?
a) F41.1
b) F41.9
c) F40.01
d) F43.10

42. 'A 60-year-old patient with COPD presents with acute bronchitis. What is the correct ICD-10-CM code?
a) J44.0
b) J44.1
c) J42
d) J20.9

43. 'A patient presents with chronic obstructive pulmonary disease with chronic respiratory failure. What is the correct ICD-10-CM code?
a) J44.9, J96.10
b) J44.9, J96.00
c) J44.1, J96.10
d) J44.1, J96.90

44. 'A 40-year-old male is diagnosed with cluster headaches. What is the correct ICD-10-CM code?
a) G44.209
b) G44.01
c) G44.009
d) G43.001

45. 'A 55-year-old male is diagnosed with Barrett's esophagus without dysplasia. What is the correct ICD-10-CM code?
a) K22.70
b) K22.710
c) K22.711
d) K22.719

46. 'A 78-year-old male presents with a stage 3 pressure ulcer of the sacrum. What is the correct ICD-10-CM code?
a) L89.152
b) L89.153
c) L89.154
d) L89.159

47. 'A 25-year-old female presents with primary infertility. What is the correct ICD-10-CM code?
a) N97.0
b) N97.1
c) N97.9
d) N97.4

48. 'A patient presents with a traumatic complete amputation of the right thumb. What is the correct ICD-10-CM **code?**
a) S68.011A
b) S68.112A
c) S68.021A
d) S68.122A

49. 'A 45-year-old female with hypothyroidism due to Hashimoto's thyroiditis is seen for follow-up. What is the correct ICD-10-CM **code?**
a) E06.3, E03.9
b) E06.9, E03.9
c) E06.3
d) E03.8

50. 'A 35-year-old patient presents with acute otitis media with spontaneous rupture of the tympanic membrane. What is the correct ICD-10-CM **code?**
a) H66.001
b) H66.002
c) H66.013
d) H66.012

51. 'A 50-year-old male presents with acute diverticulitis of the colon without perforation or abscess. What is the correct ICD-10-CM **code?**
a) K57.32
b) K57.30
c) K57.20
d) K57.90

52. 'A 60-year-old patient presents with osteoarthritis of both knees. What is the correct ICD-10-CM **code?**
a) M17.0
b) M17.11
c) M17.12
d) M17.9

53. 'A 19-year-old male presents with allergic rhinitis due to pollen. What is the correct ICD-10-CM **code?**
a) J30.1
b) J30.0
c) J30.2
d) J30.9

54. 'A patient presents with chronic allergic contact dermatitis due to nickel exposure. What is the correct ICD-10-CM **code?**
a) L23.0
b) L23.1
c) L23.2
d) L23.3

55. 'A 50-year-old male presents with gastroesophageal reflux disease without esophagitis. What is the correct ICD-10-CM **code?**
a) K21.0
b) K21.9
c) K22.70
d) K20.8

56. 'A 75-year-old female presents with severe protein-calorie malnutrition. What is the correct ICD-10-CM **code?**
a) E43
b) E44.1
c) E46
d) E44.0

57. 'A patient presents with anemia due to chronic kidney disease, stage 5. What is the correct ICD-10-CM **code?**
a) N18.5, D63.1
b) D63.1, N18.5
c) D63.8, N18.5
d) D63.0, N18.5

58. 'A 72-year-old male presents with severe aortic valve stenosis and undergoes a transcatheter aortic valve replacement (TAVR). What is the correct ICD-10-CM **code for the diagnosis?**
a) I35.0
b) I35.1
c) I35.2
d) I06.2

59. 'A 45-year-old female presents with chronic migraine with aura but without intractability. What is the correct ICD-10-CM **code?**
a) G43.109
b) G43.119
c) G43.001
d) G43.009

60. 'A 60-year-old male is diagnosed with Parkinson's disease with associated dementia. What is the correct ICD-10-CM **code?**
a) G20, F02.80
b) G21.4, F02.81
c) G20
d) F02.81

61. 'A 28-year-old female at 36 weeks gestation is diagnosed with cholestasis of pregnancy. What is the correct ICD-10-CM **code?**
a) O26.611
b) O26.612
c) O26.619
d) O26.63

62. 'A 50-year-old male presents with alcoholic cirrhosis of the liver with ascites. What is the correct ICD-10-CM **code?**
a) K70.30
b) K70.31
c) K74.60
d) K76.6

63. 'A 40-year-old patient presents with acute anterior uveitis of the left eye. What is the correct ICD-10-CM **code?**
a) H20.021
b) H20.022
c) H20.029
d) H21.529

64. 'A newborn presents with neonatal hypoglycemia due to maternal diabetes. What is the correct ICD-10-CM code?
a) P70.0
b) P70.1
c) P70.2
d) P70.9

65. 'A 65-year-old female presents with a nontraumatic subarachnoid hemorrhage from the left middle cerebral artery. What is the correct ICD-10-CM code?
a) I60.3
b) I60.2
c) I60.4
d) I60.9

66. 'A 50-year-old patient presents with an acute exacerbation of chronic bronchitis. What is the correct ICD-10-CM code?
a) J44.1
b) J42
c) J40
d) J44.9

67. 'A 72-year-old male with osteoporosis suffers a pathological fracture of the right humerus. What is the correct ICD-10-CM code?
a) M80.021A
b) M80.021D
c) M81.0
d) M80.00XA

68. 'A 35-year-old male presents with hidradenitis suppurativa of both axillae. What is the correct ICD-10-CM code?
a) L73.2
b) L73.9
c) L74.3
d) L73.1

69. 'A 55-year-old female presents with postmenopausal osteoporosis without fractures. What is the correct ICD-10-CM code?
a) M80.0AXA
b) M80.80XA
c) M81.0
d) M81.8

70. 'A 30-year-old male presents with spontaneous pneumothorax. What is the correct ICD-10-CM code?
a) J93.11
b) J93.82
c) J94.2
d) J96.01

71. 'A 40-year-old male presents with a recurrent inguinal hernia without obstruction or gangrene. What is the correct ICD-10-CM code?
a) K40.91
b) K40.90
c) K41.91
d) K41.90

72. 'A 60-year-old male is diagnosed with acute myocardial infarction of the right coronary artery. What is the correct ICD-10-CM code?
a) I21.11
b) I21.01
c) I21.02
d) I21.4

73. 'A 45-year-old male presents with malignant neoplasm of the sigmoid colon. What is the correct ICD-10-CM code?
a) C18.7
b) C18.0
c) C18.6
d) C19

74. 'A 70-year-old female presents with vertebral compression fractures due to osteoporosis. What is the correct ICD-10-CM code?
a) M80.08XA
b) M80.00XA
c) M80.9
d) M81.0

75. 'A 50-year-old male is diagnosed with lumbosacral radiculopathy. What is the correct ICD-10-CM code?
a) M54.16
b) M54.17
c) M54.15
d) M54.9

76. 'A patient presents with cellulitis of the right foot. What is the correct ICD-10-CM code?
a) L03.119
b) L03.115
c) L03.116
d) L03.113

77. 'A 75-year-old male presents with chronic venous hypertension with ulceration of the right lower leg. What is the correct ICD-10-CM code?
a) I87.319
b) I87.311
c) I87.329
d) I87.31

78. 'A 35-year-old male presents with acute otitis externa in both ears. What is the correct ICD-10-CM code?
a) H60.33
b) H60.32
c) H60.31
d) H60.39

79. 'A 55-year-old female presents with iron deficiency anemia due to chronic blood loss. What is the correct ICD-10-CM code?
a) D50.0
b) D50.8
c) D50.9
d) D51.0

80. 'A 40-year-old female presents with an ovarian cyst on the right side. What is the correct ICD-10-CM **code?**
a) N83.201
b) N83.202
c) N83.209
d) N83.291

81. 'A 20-year-old male presents with a concussion with brief loss of consciousness. What is the correct ICD-10-CM **code?**
a) S06.0X1A
b) S06.0X0A
c) S06.0X9A
d) S06.0X8A

82. 'A 60-year-old patient is diagnosed with diabetic neuropathy due to type 2 diabetes. What is the correct ICD-10-CM **code?**
a) E11.40
b) E11.42
c) E11.49
d) E11.21

83. 'A 50-year-old male is diagnosed with aortic dissection of the descending thoracic aorta. What is the correct ICD-10-CM **code?**
a) I71.03
b) I71.02
c) I71.01
d) I71.9

84. 'A 30-year-old female presents with a Bartholin's gland abscess. What is the correct ICD-10-CM **code?**
a) N75.0
b) N75.1
c) N75.8
d) N76.4

85. 'A 45-year-old female presents with interstitial cystitis with hematuria. What is the correct ICD-10-CM **code?**
a) N30.21
b) N30.20
c) N30.11
d) N30.91

ANSWERS PRACTICE TEST

1. **b) N40.1**
   'N40.1 is the correct code for benign prostatic hyperplasia with lower urinary tract symptoms, as it specifically includes both the prostate enlargement and associated urinary complaints.'

2. **a) N18.3**
   'N18.3 is the correct code because it accurately represents chronic kidney disease stage 3, which is categorized as moderate kidney dysfunction.'

3. **a) A**
   'The seventh character "A" is used for initial encounters, indicating that active treatment is being provided for the tibial fracture.'

4. **a) G44.209**
   'G44.209 is the correct code for tension-type headache, unspecified, as it falls under the category of chronic headaches without further classification.'

5. **b) E11.65**
   'E11.65 is the correct code for type 2 diabetes mellitus with hyperglycemia, as it specifies the presence of high blood sugar levels in addition to diabetes.'

6. **a) J10.1**
   'J10.1 correctly identifies influenza A with pneumonia, which falls under the category of flu-related respiratory infections caused by influenza A virus.'

7. **a) I21.01**
   'I21.01 is the correct code for an acute myocardial infarction of the anterior wall, a condition that affects the left anterior descending artery.'

8. **a) B18.2**
   'B18.2 is the correct code because it represents chronic viral hepatitis C, a long-term liver infection caused by the hepatitis C virus.'

9. **a) I15.9**
   'I15.9 is the correct code for secondary hypertension, which is high blood pressure caused by an underlying medical condition.'

10. **a) P22.1**
    'P22.1 is the correct code for transient tachypnea of the newborn, a temporary breathing difficulty commonly seen in full-term newborns.'

11. **b) K21.0**
    'K21.0 is the correct code for gastroesophageal reflux disease (GERD) with esophagitis, as it includes inflammation of the esophagus caused by acid reflux.'

12. **c) K80.12**
    'K80.12 correctly identifies acute cholecystitis with gallstones and obstruction, a condition that requires urgent medical attention.'

13. **a) A87.0**
    'A87.0 is the correct code for viral meningitis due to enterovirus, which is one of the most common causes of viral meningitis.'

14. **a) O72.0**
    'O72.0 is the correct code for postpartum hemorrhage, which refers to excessive bleeding following childbirth.'

15. **a) F20.0**

'F20.0 is the correct code for paranoid schizophrenia, a subtype of schizophrenia characterized by delusions and auditory hallucinations.'

16. **b) E11.321**

'E11.321 correctly represents mild nonproliferative diabetic retinopathy with macular edema, a common complication of diabetes affecting vision.'

17. **b) M1A.0720**

'M1A.0720 is the correct code for chronic gout with tophi in the left ankle, as it specifies both the chronic nature and presence of tophi deposits.'

18. **a) N30.10**

'N30.10 is the correct code for interstitial cystitis without hematuria, a chronic bladder condition causing pain and urinary urgency.'

19. **a) G35**

'G35 is the correct code for multiple sclerosis, a chronic neurological disease affecting the brain and spinal cord.'

20. **a) G51.0**

'G51.0 correctly identifies Bell's palsy, a sudden, temporary weakness or paralysis of the facial muscles.'

21. **b) K85.9**

'K85.9 is the correct code for acute pancreatitis without necrosis or infection, which is a common inflammatory condition of the pancreas.'

22. **a) M80.08XA**

'M80.08XA is the correct code for primary osteoporosis with a current pathological vertebral fracture, indicating that the fracture is a direct result of bone weakness.'

23. **b) J45.42**

'J45.42 is the correct code for moderate persistent asthma with status asthmaticus, which refers to a prolonged, severe asthma attack requiring immediate medical attention.'

24. **a) G21.8**

'G21.8 is the correct code for secondary Parkinsonism due to another medical condition, as it differentiates it from primary Parkinson's disease (G20).'

25. **a) S06.5X5A**

'S06.5X5A is the correct code for a traumatic subdural hemorrhage with loss of consciousness greater than 24 hours, which is classified as a severe brain injury.'

26. **a) I69.354**

'I69.354 is the correct code for left-sided hemiplegia due to an old cerebral infarction, indicating residual paralysis following a previous stroke.'

27. **a) E87.6**

'E87.6 is the correct code for hypokalemia, a condition characterized by low potassium levels in the blood, which can cause muscle weakness and cardiac arrhythmias.'

28. **a) A41.51**

'A41.51 is the correct code for sepsis due to E. coli, a bacterial bloodstream infection leading to systemic inflammation and organ dysfunction.'

29. **a) M16.11**

'M16.11 is the correct code for osteoarthritis of the right hip, as it specifies both the location and the degenerative nature of the joint disease.'

30. **a) K35.20**

'K35.20 is the correct code for acute appendicitis with perforation but without abscess, as it accurately captures the condition without additional complications.'

31. **b) I12.9, N18.4**

'I12.9 is the correct code for hypertensive chronic kidney disease without heart failure, and N18.4 specifies stage 4 chronic kidney disease.'

32. **b) O14.12**

'O14.12 is the correct code for pre-eclampsia with severe features in the second trimester, distinguishing it from mild or unspecified forms.'

33. **a) I20.0**

'I20.0 is the correct code for unstable angina, which is a form of acute coronary syndrome requiring urgent medical attention.'

34. **a) P24.00**

'P24.00 is the correct code for meconium aspiration syndrome, which can cause respiratory distress in newborns.'

35. **b) I50.21**

'I50.21 is the correct code for acute systolic heart failure, indicating left ventricular dysfunction requiring immediate treatment.'

36. **b) Z99.2**

'Z99.2 is the correct code for dialysis dependence, used alongside N18.6 for end-stage renal disease.'

37. **c) F10.239**

'F10.239 is the correct code for alcohol dependence with intoxication and withdrawal, as it accounts for all aspects of the patient's condition.'

38. **b) O24.414**

'O24.414 is the correct code for gestational diabetes, diet controlled, in the second trimester, aligning with trimester-specific coding rules.'

39. **a) A**

'The seventh character "A" indicates an initial encounter, meaning active treatment is still ongoing for the femur fracture.'

40. **b) G51.0**

'G51.0 is the correct code for Bell's palsy, a condition that causes temporary paralysis of facial muscles.'

41. **b) F41.9**

'F41.9 is the correct code for generalized anxiety disorder, which includes chronic excessive worry and stress-related symptoms.'

42. **a) J44.0**

'J44.0 is the correct code for COPD with acute lower respiratory infection, covering both the chronic lung disease and current infection.'

43. **a) J44.9, J96.10**

'J44.9 represents chronic obstructive pulmonary disease (COPD), while J96.10 specifies chronic respiratory failure with hypoxia.'

44. **b) G44.01**

'G44.01 is the correct code for cluster headaches, a severe neurological disorder characterized by recurring attacks of pain.'

45. **a) K22.70**

'K22.70 is the correct code for Barrett's esophagus without dysplasia, distinguishing it from cases with confirmed cellular changes.'

46. **b) L89.153**

'L89.153 is the correct code for a stage 3 pressure ulcer of the sacrum, indicating a deep wound affecting the fat layer.'

47. **a) N97.0**
   'N97.0 is the correct code for primary female infertility, referring to the inability to conceive without prior pregnancies.'

48. **a) S68.011A**
   'S68.011A is the correct code for a traumatic complete amputation of the right thumb, specifying laterality and encounter type.'

49. **c) E06.3**
   'E06.3 is the correct code for Hashimoto's thyroiditis, a common cause of hypothyroidism, without needing an additional hypothyroidism code.'

50. **d) H66.012**
   'H66.012 is the correct code for acute otitis media with spontaneous rupture of the tympanic membrane in the left ear.'

51. **b) K57.30**
   'K57.30 is the correct code for acute diverticulitis of the large intestine without perforation or abscess.'

52. **a) M17.0**
   'M17.0 is the correct code for bilateral primary osteoarthritis of the knees, indicating a degenerative joint disease in both knees.'

53. **a) J30.1**
   'J30.1 is the correct code for allergic rhinitis due to pollen, commonly known as hay fever.'

54. **a) L23.0**
   'L23.0 is the correct code for allergic contact dermatitis due to nickel, a common cause of skin reactions.'

55. **b) K21.9**
   'K21.9 is the correct code for gastroesophageal reflux disease without esophagitis, distinguishing it from cases with inflammation.'

56. **a) E43**
   'E43 is the correct code for severe protein-calorie malnutrition, a life-threatening condition often seen in elderly or chronically ill patients.'

57. **b) D63.1, N18.5**
   'D63.1 is the correct code for anemia due to chronic kidney disease, and N18.5 specifies stage 5 CKD.'

58. **a) I35.0**
   'I35.0 is the correct code for nonrheumatic aortic valve stenosis, which is the most common indication for transcatheter aortic valve replacement (TAVR).'

59. **a) G43.109**
   'G43.109 is the correct code for chronic migraine with aura without intractability, as it specifies the presence of aura but not persistent migraine attacks.'

60. **a) G20, F02.80**
   'G20 represents Parkinson's disease, and F02.80 indicates associated dementia without behavioral disturbance, which is common in later stages of Parkinson's.'

61. **c) O26.619**
   'O26.619 is the correct code for cholestasis of pregnancy, unspecified trimester, as it accounts for pregnancy-related liver dysfunction.'

62. **b) K70.31**
   'K70.31 correctly represents alcoholic cirrhosis of the liver with ascites, distinguishing it from cases without fluid accumulation.'

63. **b) H20.022**
   'H20.022 is the correct code for acute anterior uveitis of the left eye, which refers to inflammation affecting the front part of the uveal tract.'

64. **b) P70.1**

   'P70.1 is the correct code for neonatal hypoglycemia due to maternal diabetes, distinguishing it from transient hypoglycemia.'

65. **c) I60.4**

   'I60.4 is the correct code for a nontraumatic subarachnoid hemorrhage from the left middle cerebral artery, a common location for aneurysmal rupture.'

66. **a) J44.1**

   'J44.1 is the correct code for an acute exacerbation of chronic bronchitis, indicating a worsening of COPD symptoms.'

67. **a) M80.021A**

   'M80.021A is the correct code for osteoporosis with a pathological fracture of the right humerus, specifying an initial encounter for treatment.'

68. **a) L73.2**

   'L73.2 is the correct code for hidradenitis suppurativa, a chronic skin condition affecting hair follicles, typically in the axillae and groin.'

69. **c) M81.0**

   'M81.0 is the correct code for postmenopausal osteoporosis without fractures, differentiating it from cases with pathological fractures.'

70. **a) J93.11**

   'J93.11 is the correct code for spontaneous pneumothorax, meaning a collapsed lung occurring without an external injury.'

71. **b) K40.90**

   'K40.90 is the correct code for a unilateral recurrent inguinal hernia without obstruction or gangrene, distinguishing it from bilateral cases.'

72. **a) I21.11**

   'I21.11 is the correct code for an acute myocardial infarction of the right coronary artery, which is a common site for heart attacks.'

73. **c) C18.6**

   'C18.6 is the correct code for a malignant neoplasm of the sigmoid colon, one of the most frequently diagnosed colorectal cancers.'

74. **a) M80.08XA**

   'M80.08XA is the correct code for vertebral compression fractures due to osteoporosis, specifying an initial encounter for active treatment.'

75. **b) M54.17**

   'M54.17 is the correct code for lumbosacral radiculopathy, a condition involving nerve root compression in the lower spine.'

76. **c) L03.116**

   'L03.116 is the correct code for cellulitis of the right foot, indicating a bacterial skin infection with localized inflammation.'

77. **b) I87.311**

   'I87.311 is the correct code for chronic venous hypertension with ulceration of the right lower leg, differentiating it from stasis dermatitis or edema alone.'

78. **a) H60.33**

   'H60.33 is the correct code for acute otitis externa in both ears, specifying a bilateral outer ear infection.'

79. **a) D50.0**

   'D50.0 is the correct code for iron deficiency anemia due to chronic blood loss, a common result of gastrointestinal bleeding or heavy menstrual cycles.'

80. **a) N83.201**

   'N83.201 is the correct code for a right ovarian cyst, indicating an unspecified type of cyst in the right ovary.'

81. **a) S06.0X1A**

   'S06.0X1A is the correct code for a concussion with brief loss of consciousness, distinguishing it from prolonged or unspecified loss of consciousness.'

82. **a) E11.40**

   'E11.40 is the correct code for type 2 diabetes with diabetic neuropathy, specifying nerve damage related to diabetes without further complications.'

83. **a) I71.03**

   'I71.03 is the correct code for an aortic dissection of the descending thoracic aorta, which can lead to severe cardiovascular complications.'

84. **a) N75.0**

   'N75.0 is the correct code for a Bartholin's gland abscess, an infected cyst in the vaginal area requiring drainage or antibiotics.'

85. **a) N30.21**

   'N30.21 is the correct code for interstitial cystitis with hematuria, differentiating it from cases without blood in the urine.'

EXTRA CONTENT ACCESS

D ear Valued Reader,
Embarking on this book marks the start of a rewarding journey, and we are privileged to accompany you. As a token of our gratitude, we have prepared a special set of additional resources for you:

DIGITAL COPY OF THIS BOOK to have with you at all times for revision whenever and wherever you want.

DIRECT CONTACT for assistance or clarifications, ensuring continuous support in your preparation.

COMPLETE VIDEO COURSE: Dive deeper into essential topics like ICD-10-CM coding, medical billing errors, and revenue cycle processes through a professionally designed video course tailored for medical coding professionals specializing in diagnosis coding.

3000 MEDICAL TERMS FLASHCARDS:

- **2500 Medical Terms** covering Surgery, Emergency Medicine, and Anesthesiology.
- **50 Flashcards featuring Real-World Case Studies** illustrating medical conditions and treatments for practical application in billing and coding.
- **600 Medical Terms** *with pictures*

Do you want more?

EXTRA RESOURCE OF YOUR CHOICE: Enhance Your Learning Journey!

We are excited to offer you one of the following **additional resources**—completely free of charge! Just send us an email and let us know which resource you'd like to receive. You can choose between:

- **Medical Billing and Coding**: *Are you working in healthcare administration or planning to enhance your billing and coding skills?* This guide covers the essential processes, compliance regulations, and technologies needed for accurate and efficient healthcare billing practices.
- **CPC Study Guide**: *Are you preparing for the Certified Professional Coder (CPC) exam or looking to refine your coding expertise?* This study guide provides exam-focused strategies, practice questions, and detailed explanations to help you succeed in the certification process.
- **CPT Professional Mastery Workbook**: *Do you work in clinical coding and want to master CPT coding?* This guide provides a comprehensive overview of procedural coding standards, updates, and practical exercises to strengthen your expertise in medical procedure and service coding.
- **HCPCS Level II Coding Workbook:** *Are you involved in medical billing or outpatient services and need to strengthen your understanding of HCPCS Level II codes?* This workbook provides a clear, hands-on approach to mastering billing supplies, services, and durable medical equipment coding. With practical exercises, real-world scenarios, and access to a full video course, it's the perfect tool to enhance your skills in billing accuracy and reimbursement optimization.

How to Claim Your Resource

Simply email us, and include the following details: your name, your profession or area of interest, and the title of the resource you'd like to receive. **This is a gift from us to you, with no strings attached!** There will be *no subscriptions to newsletters or mailing lists*; we offer these materials purely to support your professional development.

Unlock your exclusive study materials
Simply scan the QR code below to unlock everything instantly.

Need help or have a question?

Write to us at: **info.testbookreader@gmail.com**

With gratitude,
Rory George

Thank you!